W9-AOD-770

Keep Your Voice Healthy

Keep Your Voice Healthy

A GUIDE TO THE INTELLIGENT USE AND CARE OF THE SPEAKING AND SINGING VOICE

by Friedrich S. Brodnitz, M.D.

Introduction by Olin Downes

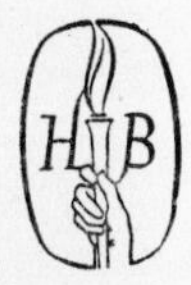

HARPER & BROTHERS PUBLISHERS NEW YORK

KEEP YOUR VOICE HEALTHY

Printed in the United States of America

FIRST EDITION

H-C

Library of Congress catalog card number: 53-7725

To the Memory of

MANUEL GARCIA (1805-1906)

Singer, Teacher, Scientist

who gave to medicine the laryngeal mirror
and opened a new era
in the study of the human voice

Contents

Illustrations

Acknowledgments

To write a popular book on a medical subject is impossible without the help of a great many people.

First of all, science is, by its very nature, a co-operative undertaking. The doctor who writes for his colleagues in medical journals or books quotes his sources in numerous footnotes. In popular writing this technique would be confusing to the reader. But I want to say that all the workers who, by their original thoughts and research, developed the science of the human voice and speech are, in a deeper sense, the co-authors of this book.

Thanks are due to my patients and to the students of my lectures and courses on voice problems who, through their questions, helped to test and clarify the terms, definitions and explanations I had to give on many occasions. Their willingness to listen and to partake in discussions of a sometimes rather involved subject has encouraged me to write in nontechnical language but without the oversimplification that is the danger of popular medical literature.

A number of friends, colleagues, scientists have helped me immensely by their generous and selfless assistance in putting this book together:

Helmuth Nathan, M.D., of New York City, contributed the drawings;

Emil Froeschels, M.D., of New York City, read the manuscript and gave valuable criticism and advice;

Gordon E. Peterson, Ph.D., of Murray Hill, New Jersey, and R. R. Garcia, of New York City, both of the Bell Telephone Laboratories, supplied photographs of the vocal cords:

Joel J. Pressman, M.D., of Beverly Hills, California (and the American Medical Association as publishers) permitted the use of illustrations from his paper on the vocal cords in the *Archives of Otolaryngology*, 1942;

Deso A. Weiss, M.D., of New York City, contributed his scheme of the mutational disturbances of the voice from the proceedings of the VIII International Speech and Voice Therapy Conference, Amsterdam, 1950;

G. Panconcelli-Calzia, M.D., of Hamburg, Germany, put at my disposal a copy of his otherwise unobtainable book *Historical Data on Phonetics*;

Johann Urzidil, of New York City, translated the concluding poem by Goethe.

To these men, I wish to extend my most sincere thanks for a co-operation that was given in the spirit of the brotherhood of science.

Finally, I want to acknowledge with appreciation: the permission, given by the publishers of *Time* Magazine, to use an anecdote from an article on David Sarnoff (July, 1952); the permission, given by the publishers of *Musical Opinion*, London to use a quotation from Sterling MacKinlay's articles on Manuel Garcia (1948).

F. S. B.

New York City
March, 1953

Introduction by Olin Downes

THE LITERATURE ABOUT THE SINGING AND SPEAKING VOICE IS as voluminous as it is bewildering. Confusion reigns in this field almost in multiple ratio to the number of theories, doctrines, superstitions that are propounded.

A very few works by masters of the vocal art stand out for their knowledge and authority. But even there wide disagreement exists. The Garcia method, as set forth in his justly famous *Mémoire sur la voix humaine*, differs from that of Lamperti or Lombardi who trained Caruso.

The fact that even the masters disagree shows that there are different approaches to the fundamental truth, and also, perhaps, points to the fact that no two voices, temperaments and physical organisms are the same. The success of a vocal teacher with his pupils, the success of these pupils themselves with the public, seem often to be a matter of chance: a teacher has a system of pedagogy which, by a stroke of good luck, fits certain voices well; or a singer has the rare good luck of possessing a voice of inherently fine quality and a vocal mechanism which works naturally and instinctively in the right way.

There appears to be no norm, no single reliable method to which all competent teachers and singers subscribe. Legions of vocal students wander from teacher to teacher in search of the vocal truth. There have even been singers of reputation who became obsessed by a Freudian doubt of their tone production and then embarked upon a course of ill-advised voice experiments which cost them their careers.

The professional who uses the speaking voice as his most important tool is confronted with a similar problem. As a rule, nobody ever tells him anything about the instrument he uses constantly. In the training of teachers, ministers, actors and other professionals little attention is paid to the problems of the speaking voice.

Dr. Brodnitz's book is based upon firsthand knowledge of the vocal organs and the way they operate. His approach to voice production stems from an understanding of artistic problems as well as from an extensive experience with the working conditions of singers and public speakers.

He advocates no "method" of a narrowly restricted sort. His central premise is the recognition of scientific principles from which any sound vocal practice must proceed.

Indispensable to the understanding of the voice and its problems are the chapters on the hygiene of the vocal organs, medical treatment of their diseases, disturbances of voice and speech which can be remedied, discussed in nontechnical language calculated to inform anyone who is interested in this subject.

And the subject is one which concerns all who desire to develop more beautiful and intelligent ways of using man's main instrument of communication with his fellows—the voice and its magic.

Keep Your Voice Healthy

I. *You and Your Voice*

In the autumn of 1854, on one of those exquisite sunny days when Paris is at its best, a man stood in the courtyard of the Palais Royal in the midst of the stream of people who used this passage before the great boulevards were created in the reign of Napoleon III.

But the man paid no attention to the palace which had seen Richelieu, the Revolution, the Empire and now the Orleans. He had no eye for the elegant stores, the coffeehouses with their little tables and the crowd of busy Parisians, idle do-nothings, admiring strangers. He stood there in the midst of the jostling crowd with the expression of a man who has suddenly been hit by an idea.

Manuel Garcia, the most famous singing teacher of his time, then in his fiftieth year, had never been satisfied to give lessons to young artists. He had known the musical world from childhood on. The son of a great singer of Spanish birth and international reputation he had seen the backstages of all Europe. In 1828 he even accompanied his father to New York where they presented with *Figaro* the first stage performance of an opera in this city while Mozart's librettist Lorenzo da Ponte sat in the audience.

Shortly afterward he lost his voice, which kept him from further public appearances. But out of this crisis came the determination to learn more about the human voice. Within a few years he became one of the best known teachers, first in Paris and later in London to whom students of all countries flocked.

He studied all available books on anatomy and function of the vocal organs. He took part in anatomy classes, dissected human and animal bodies until he knew more about the voice box than most doctors.

But all research did not satisfy him. Dead organs cannot answer questions about their function in life. Nobody had yet *seen* the human vocal cords in action, in speaking and singing. While the professionals did not pay much attention, this medical amateur had racked his brain to find the solution to the problem of making voice visible.

As it so often happens in medicine, the determined outsider had the imagination and the good luck to have the creative idea. While he stood in the Palais Royal it suddenly occurred to him: Why not try it with mirrors.

He rushed to the store of Charrière, a maker of medical instruments and found there a small dental mirror, left over as a failure from an exhibition in London. He bought the mirror for six francs and went back to his room to start his experiment without delay. Standing near the window he flashed the sunlight with a large hand mirror into his mouth while he introduced with the other hand the small dental mirror deep into his throat.

With a stroke of good luck he chose at the first attempt the right angles for both mirrors and suddenly saw his own vocal cords, reflected first in the dental and from there in the large mirror.

As he described it later to his pupil Sterling MacKinlay: "There before my very eyes appeared the glottis (the space between the vocal cords) wide open. . . . So astounded was I that I sank back into my chair and for several minutes remained there without moving, aghast, dumbfounded. I was the first human being to see the larynx of a living man and that man myself. Slowly I recovered from the shock and rose again to my feet. Once more I placed the dentist's mirror in the correct position, then with the larger mirror directed the ray of sunlight into the mouth. . . . Again the vocal cords made their appearance in the little circle of glass.

"Next I experimented in emitting various single notes, an upward scale, a downward one, an arpeggio, the registers. Then a laugh, a cry, all sorts of queer sounds, animal imitations, whatever came into my head. On and on I went, almost like a madman, until the voice was so completely tired that I had to remain silent for a long, long time."

In telling you the events of this exciting hour in some detail we have been guided by this reason:

The invention of the laryngeal mirror by Manuel Garcia marks the birth hour of the science of the human voice. When Garcia died in 1906, one hundred and one years old, doctors, scientists, singing teachers of the whole world united in a tribute to a man who had given them the tool for countless new studies, for diagnosing and treating diseases of the larynx.

Again, in 1954, the centenary of this great discovery will be remembered by speech and voice therapists, physicians and singing teachers.

True, from time of antiquity on, men have tried to understand the miracle of the human voice. And after Garcia, generations of workers have labored to compile a vast literature on vocal problems.

But that does not diminish the importance of the man who, in the true sense of the word, threw light into a hidden part of the human body and taught us to understand by seeing what makes us speak and sing.

But there is another, and more personal, reason which makes it, in our opinion, so appropriate to begin this book with Manuel Garcia. In all his years of teaching Garcia has fought for the idea that the professional user of the voice should *know* something about the nature and function of his instrument. In later years, this conviction even put him in the paradoxical position of arguing with one of the greatest throat specialists of his time about the value of scientific knowledge for the artist and professional who lives by his voice.

When Sir Morel Mackenzie expressed his doubts about the benefit a voice student could derive in his practical handling of the voice from a study of structure and function of the vocal organs, Garcia replied: "I still believe that some exact scientific notions on the formation and the action of the vocal organs would be more useful than hurtful to the rising singer."

This, then, is the basic conviction of this book which is addressed not only to the singer but to everybody who needs voice for success in his pursuits. Unless you work only with your hands, voice is your tool. Much more depends on the quality, the character, the handling of your voice than most people realize. People in all walks of life are hired because of the attractiveness or persuasiveness of their voices. You close a deal, you acquit as juror a defendant, you vote for a politician, you follow your conscience after a sermon, you even marry because a voice has captivated you with just the right degree of genuine conviction, of true pathos or cool explanation, of moral zeal or tender affection.

You influence people as often with your voice as they impress you with theirs. And you have only to remember your last laryngitis to understand what a handicap even a temporary impairment of the voice means in every moment of the day.

Knowledge is necessary to understand the functions of our voice, to guard its health and to handle any danger that threatens to destroy it. This book was written because, as a rule, nobody told us anything about the most widely used of all instruments.

To illustrate the degree of uncertainty about the most basic facts, so common even in highly trained vocal performers, we should like to tell you an experience which revealed dramatically the need for better information. Years ago, a singer with considerable experience said during an examination: "Doctor, for a long time I have meant to ask somebody who knows: are the vocal cords suspended vertically or horizontally?" Before answering him we tried to find out what his conception of voice production was. It turned out that he had some vague notions about vertically placed bands, exposed in the windpipe to the air stream and made to sing in some miraculous way.

We still refused to believe that this experience could be generalized and began to ask singers, actors, teachers, ministers the same question. We quickly realized that the right answer: that the cords are horizontally suspended, was given only by a few, and then mostly by good luck. When finally a well-known singing teacher confessed with considerable embarrassment that he knew next to nothing about the structure and function of the vocal organs, it became clear that something is wrong with the training of people who use the speaking or singing voice in their work.

Modern education has abolished the authoritarian approach of bygone days. We prefer the student who does not just imitate the teacher but asks questions, demands explanations, understands thoroughly before he accepts offered knowledge.

But singers and other professionals of the voice are still trained like seals who learn by constant obedient repetition of motions, praised when successful, scolded when not responsive, but never dignified with an explanation. Actors, teachers, ministers are taught the technique of free and impressive speech but they learn little about the nature and the care of their voice.

In many lectures to groups of students in music schools and seminars, in courses for adults of all walks of life, we always found great eagerness to acquire a basic knowledge in this neglected field.

Some teachers were enthusiastic, others objected. They felt that speaking and singing is a body function which should be instinctive. They believed that too much knowledge might upset the balance of this instinctive function. They even were afraid that by lifting the vocal process into the light of consciousness the singer or speaker could develop new fears and apprehensions in addition to the many that already upset him.

With Manuel Garcia we refuse to believe that knowledge will hurt. If you ever saw the now classical film of Walt Disney's *Snow White* you will remember the scene when Snow White on her flight from the witch through the dark woods finally collapses in a clearing with a circle of burning eyes surrounding her. At that moment the sun rises, revealing harmless rabbits where we expected to encounter wild and dangerous animals.

Using the vocal organs, that are hidden away in the dark recesses of our body, we are too easily the prey of the fears and anxieties that obscurity breeds. Not all wild animals can be turned into bunnies. Some dangers to the voice, as we shall see, are quite real. But the bright sunlight of knowledge will help us to separate real dangers from imagined ones, to interpret correctly sensations of all kinds in our vocal organs, to understand the mechanics of proper function and the consequences of abuse, to prevent damage and to co-operate sensibly when help is needed.

For whom was this book written? For anybody who uses the speaking or singing voice in his day's work. It is not addressed to singers alone (although we shall discuss their problems at length). Artistic singing is the highest and most specialized form of a body function which we all use in countless pursuits of life. Voice is as important to the saleslady behind the counter, to the teacher in front of his class, to the lawyer who addresses a jury, as it is to the singer. This book intends to speak to all of them.

In writing this book we intended to fill a gap in the existing literature. The doctor, the speech therapist can turn to the many books and papers written by scientists for scientists.

Following a tradition which has made science much too exclusive, these publications speak a language which only experts can understand. They would be of no use for you.

Many books were written for the general public on improvement of elocution, speech making, singing technique, enrichment of vocabulary, polishing of speaking style.

But there is a need for a book that gives to everybody who is interested in the human voice the extract of our knowledge of function and care of our vocal organs.

Teachers of all kinds—teachers of singers and actors, instructors in training centers for all groups of professions that employ voice as a medium of communication—might welcome a book that refreshens their knowledge of the voice and helps to answer the questions of their students.

Books of factual information are particularly important for those who live away from the larger cities where scientific libraries, courses, teachers are available. The preaching minister in the village parish, the teacher in the one-class school, the small-town singer and many others depend on books if they need help with their vocal problems.

Finally, the book was written for everybody who experiences troubles with his own voice. Not that a book alone can be sufficient as a substitute for the doctor. But, at least, it can be a guide to an understanding of the prevention, the causes, the mechanism and the treatment of voice disorders.

Voice disturbances are experienced in all walks of life. Anybody with experience in treating voice patients can easily draw up a long list of typical situations. We shall meet them in all chapters of this book. To mention just a few:

The salesman who gets hoarse every day after a few hours of talking;

The secretary who could not get the better job because of her "unpleasant" voice;

The teacher who feared for the loss of his livelihood because of prolonged spells of "laryngitis";

The minister with the "clergyman's throat";

The politician whose voice breaks down in every election campaign;

The student who is tortured by stuttering;

The clubwoman who cannot be heard beyond the tenth row of the lecture hall;

The singer who develops nodes of the vocal cords;

The actor who is plagued by too many colds.

One could go on like this for a long time without exhausting the possibilities and realities of voice disorders. Most of these troubles are preventable, can be avoided by better knowledge of the proper use and care of the voice and of the possibilities of help in times of danger.

At this point a few remarks might be in order about the limitations of this book. It is not a medical textbook for the scientifically trained. To write on a medical subject for the general public involves the difficult task of selection and, sometimes, simplification of material.

The expert who should happen to glance through this book might miss details or problems he considers especially important. And he might object to a somewhat simplified explanation of a subject, the complexity of which he knows only too well.

If you, the reader, are stimulated by this book to look for more extensive knowledge in our field you will find at the end a small selection of books and medical papers for recommended reading. As it happens to everybody who goes into the depth of a science you will then see the question marks multiply. But you will be compensated for this loss in simplicity by the fascination which problems and unsolved riddles hold for the true scientist.

To leave out all unnecessary ballast we have limited the quotations of sources to the mentioning of a few names connected with important findings in our field. In scientific writing tradition and respect for the work of others requires careful documentation of every contribution to the subject under discussion with the result that sometimes the footnotes take up more space than the original work of the writer.

This book means to present to you the up-to-date knowledge about the human voice in easy-understandable terms. Scientific footnotes would only scare you away and are therefore omitted. But it should be understood that everybody who writes on a medical subject stands on the shoulders of many workers, famous and modest ones, who contributed their share to our science.

Finally, this is a doctor's book. In a specialty that is relatively young, the frontiers are not yet rigidly fixed. The doctor or the speech and voice therapist who works in this field has to know something about a number of subjects: anatomy, physiology, nose and throat diseases, psychiatry and psychology, physics and music. At the same time he has to respect certain limits to his work. He should not try to replace the experienced teacher of artistic singing or professional speaking. Doctor and teacher should work as a team, each knowing what the other can do for his ward, and realizing where the limits of his own work are. This book, a doctor's book, will stop where the professional training of the singing or speaking voice begins.

Even with these reservations, the ground to be covered will be large enough. By reading this book you will come to a better understanding of the structure and the function of the organs we use in the production of voice and speech. Having thus laid a foundation of facts that cover the normal voice, we shall then turn to the medical problems that concern the vocal organs: hygiene of the voice, self-treatment of colds, examination by the doctor and medical treatment of the vocal organs. Finally, the disturbances of the singing and speaking voice will be taken up.

Medical terms are, to a certain extent, unavoidable. They will be explained when first used. If, at later encounters, you find that the meaning of a term has slipped your memory the index will guide you back to the first definition.

In starting you on this conducted tour we like to think of you as one of the students with whom we have discussed problems of the human voice in lectures and courses. From them came the first encouragement to write down what we tried to teach. We hope that this book will give you the information you wanted when you decided to read it.

II. *The Vocal Organs*

ANY DISCUSSION OF A MEDICAL SUBJECT BEGINS WITH A DESCRIPTION of the body structures involved. As long as the knowledge of the human body was limited to the visible exterior, medicine remained a mixture of superstitions, speculative theories, witchcraft and magic traditions. Anatomy, the science of the normal human body, gained by dissection and study of organs and structures, opened the way to a real understanding of body functions and to a scientific approach to the treatment of disease.

The study of medicine begins with an intensive course in human anatomy. The mature doctor returns constantly to his anatomy books for revival and improvement of his anatomical understanding and even the lay reader cannot acquire real insight into the workings of any part of the body without the possession of a few fundamental facts about anatomy.

This poses a problem for the writer of medical books for lay readers. Anatomy is not popular; it is a dry subject and a poor start for a book that tries to encourage the reader by attractive presentation of an interesting material. The medical writer is not in the happy position of the novelist who begins with a dramatic scene and then proceeds to build up the necessary background of his story by flashbacks.

Medicine speaks a language of its own, using a multitude of

names and terms, describing structures, organs, functions, disturbances, and a certain minimum of "basic" language will be indispensable if we want to talk intelligently to you about the subject of this book.

Therefore, we shall have to ask your forbearance for a few pages of anatomical information about our vocal organs. We shall make it as brief as possible, avoiding the medical lingo wherever feasible.

In this connection another difficulty arises. Some parts of the body, although hidden from sight, are known to everybody, like the heart, the lungs, the stomach. For them, words exist in every language and no medical names need to be used to discuss them. Others are more or less unknown outside of the medical profession, yet fulfill important functions. Do you know, for instance, that you have a talus? Most probably not, although it is an important bone of your foot.

The vocal organs occupy a kind of a linguistic middle ground. We all know—and can name them in plain English—that we have a nose, throat, voice box, vocal cords, windpipe, lungs. The diaphragm and the sinuses have kept their medical names in English, French, Italian, but the terms have become part of everyday language. But if we proceed to the inner parts of the nose or the voice box we have to use medical terms.

There shall be few. We shall explain them to you as we meet them, use them as sparingly as possible and shall try altogether not to bore you if we can help it.

The most important single feature about the vocal organs is the curious fact that none of them was originally designed by creation for the production of speech and voice. All animal life depends on a constant supply of oxygen. Fishes get it by straining oxygen from the water through the gills. Millions of years back in the course of evolution, animals began to leave water, and amphibians and mammals made their appearance. To get oxygen from the air they developed lungs, connected with the outside by pipe lines from openings in the head. Noses owe their formation to the necessity of securing the vital transport of air to the lungs while the mouth is filled with food to be chewed. Even the voice box came into being not for the production of voice which is a rather late achievement of the higher mammals. It began as a safety valve to protect the lungs of amphibians while submerged against the choking penetration of water.

Respiration, the exchange of air between the outside and the lungs, is the primary purpose of all vocal organs—with the exception of the mouth which is the intake part of the digestive system too. Voice and speech have been superimposed on the organs of respiration as a kind of glorious afterthought of nature. The lungs, in addition to their function as receivers of oxygen, became bellows which blow air against the vocal cords. The cords were transformed into a musical instrument. Throat, mouth and nose became resonating chambers to step up the volume of sound and modify voice into the richness of the spoken word.

Since these two functions—respiration and voice—are so intimately connected, the logical way to explain to you the anatomy of the vocal organs is by tracing the course of air through the *respiratory tract*. By this term we describe all structures which form the pathway of inhaled air: nose, throat, voice box, windpipe, bronchi, lungs.

Air can enter the body in two ways, through the nose or through the mouth. If we breathe quietly—for instance sitting down and reading this book—we keep our mouth closed and inhale through the nose. The air enters the nose by way of the nostrils and travels through the nose to reach the throat. If you look at Fig. 1 which shows a cross section through the head near the mid-line you will be surprised by the size of the *nose*. You will notice that most of it is buried inside the head, and that what we commonly call our nose is just a projecting roof over the entrance to it. The nose is

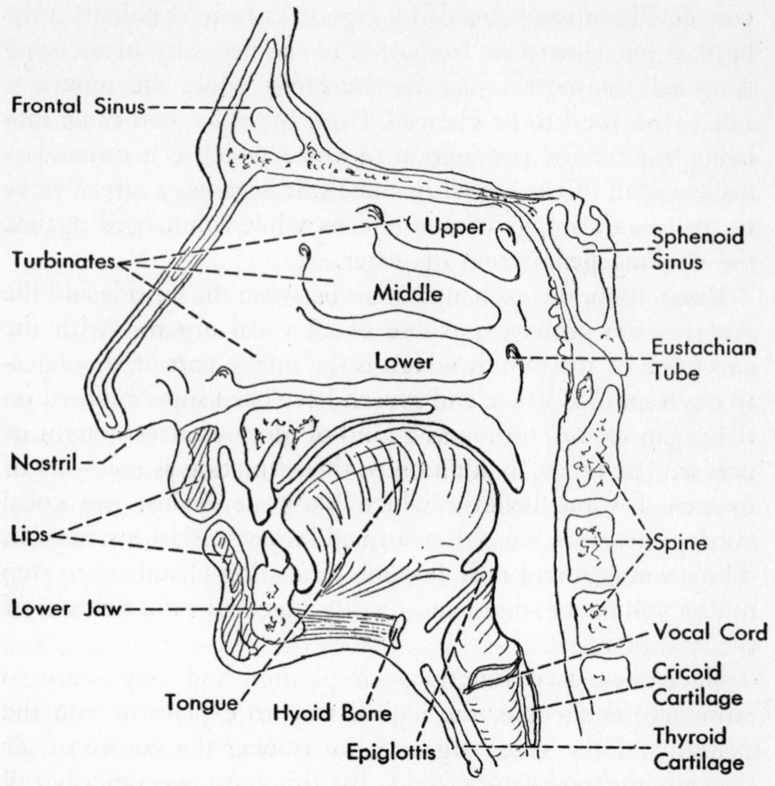

FIG. 1. Cross Section of Head and Neck

divided into two cavities, separated by a partition, the nasal *septum* the anterior rim of which you can feel between the nostrils.

We are guilty already of using medical language and supposing that you are familiar with the anatomical terms of direction. If we doctors "condescend" to give explanations at all to our patients we slip only too often into our own language which we have spoken for many years but that is so much Chinese to everybody else. So we better explain: anterior means the front end of a structure, posterior the rear.

Two points of the body can be related to each other by saying that one is anterior (or posterior) to the other one. Anything nearer to an imaginary vertical plane through the middle of the body is called medial, while points farther away from it are described as lateral. The ears, for instance, are lateral of the face, the nose medial of the eyes, the nostrils are the anterior openings of the nose through which the air travels posteriorly until it reaches the throat.

Using our newly acquired terminology we can now say that the nasal septum lies in the medial plane of the head and that the two nasal cavities are lateral of it. The cross section of the head in Fig. 1 was done slightly lateral of the mid-line. What you look at is the outer or lateral wall of the nose, and you will be impressed or confused by the complexity of the structures. Actually it is very simple. It is just the old engineering principle—used for instance in our radiators—of providing maximum surface in a cramped space by folding.

You will notice three crests, projecting like the blunt edges of a clam shell. They are the *turbinates*—the Latin word for shell—decreasing in size from the bottom to the top. The recesses under the turbinates are called *meatuses*. The middle meatus—under the middle turbinate—is a strategic spot because most of the sinuses drain there into the nose. The nasal *sinuses* are bony cavities which are connected by openings with the nasal cavities. We have four pairs of them. The largest one, the *maxillary sinus* or antrum occupies the region of the cheek, above the upper teeth and the palate and below the eyes. The *frontal sinuses* are in the forehead, above the eyes, separated from each other by a thin bony partition. Between the maxillary and frontal sinuses lies a group of small cells—near the inner angle of the eyes—called *ethmoid cells*. Finally a pair of sinuses—called *sphenoids*—is buried deep in the skull, above and behind the roof of the nose.

On the cross section of Fig. 1 you see the frontal and sphenoid sinuses, while the maxillary sinus and the ethmoid cells are hidden behind the lateral wall of the nose on which you look.

As everybody knows, the sinuses can cause a lot of trouble. But do not ask us what their function is. Nobody has yet found out. Even their role as resonating chambers for the voice is extremely doubtful, and all theories about "directing" the voice into one of the sinuses—still used by some teachers—are definitely without scientific basis.

The openings of the sinuses into the nasal cavities are hidden in deep recesses and too small to permit effective passage of sound waves into the sinuses. And even the filling of one or more of the larger sinuses with pus or polyps changes the sound of the voice surprisingly little.

All structures of the nose, sinuses and of the whole respiratory tract down to the bronchi are lined by *mucous membranes*. As the name implies, they are constantly covered by a thin layer of mucus or phlegm produced by countless tiny glands. This blanket of mucus is kept on the move by the action of microscopically small hairlike projections of the cells of the surface, called *cilia*. In the nose, their movement is directed toward the rear—the throat, in the windpipe and bronchi upward toward the throat.

Since the mucus not only lubricates all surfaces of the respiratory tract but catches dust, dirt, germs from the air, the ciliary action becomes part of the important self-cleaning mechanism which protects the health of the vocal cords, bronchi and lungs. Caught on the mucous membranes, impurities of the air we inhale travel slowly to the rear of the nose into the throat where they are disposed off into the stomach by swallowing to be destroyed there by the acid of the digestive fluids. If the membranes have to work overtime as they often do in polluted city air we notice the appearance of mucus in our throat and call it *postnasal drip*, a bugaboo with our patients but actually a sign that our nose is on the job guarding the health of the respiratory organs.

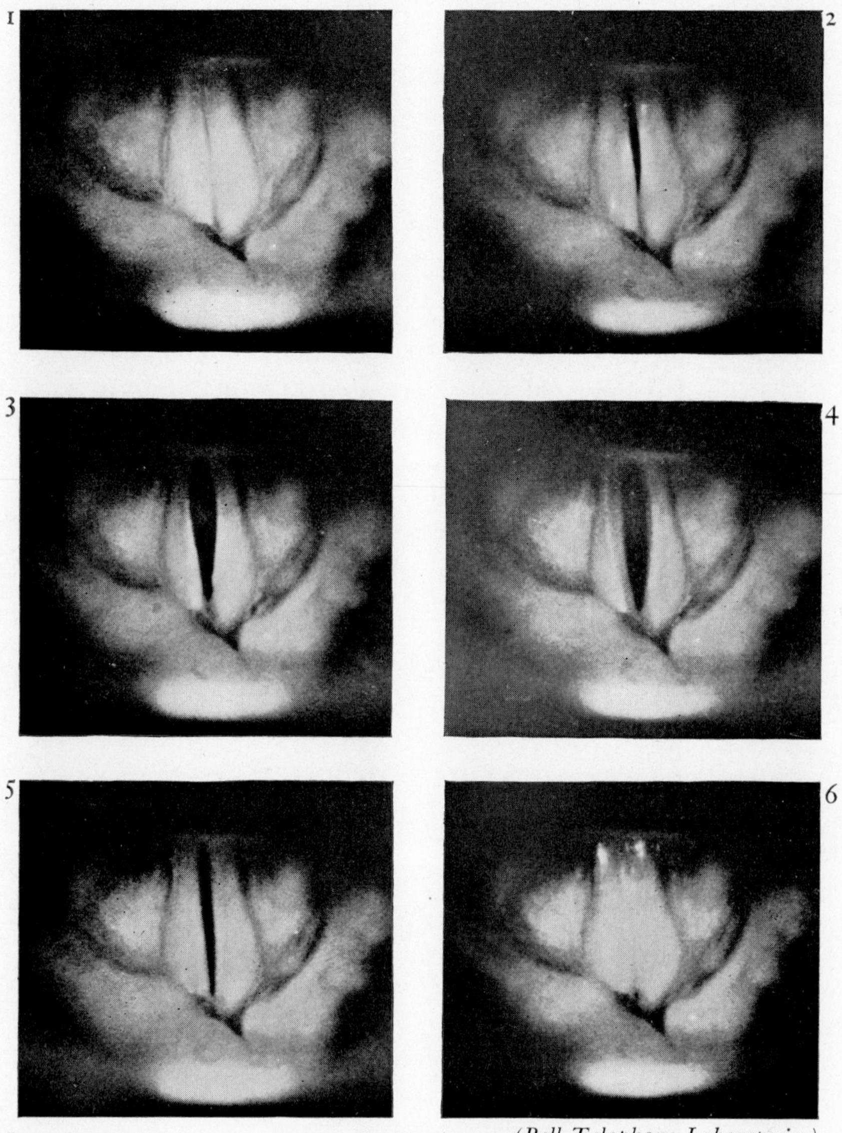

(Bell Telephone Laboratories)

PLATE I. Vibration of Vocal Cords

The photographs show six stages of one full cycle of vibration of the cords while singing c^1.

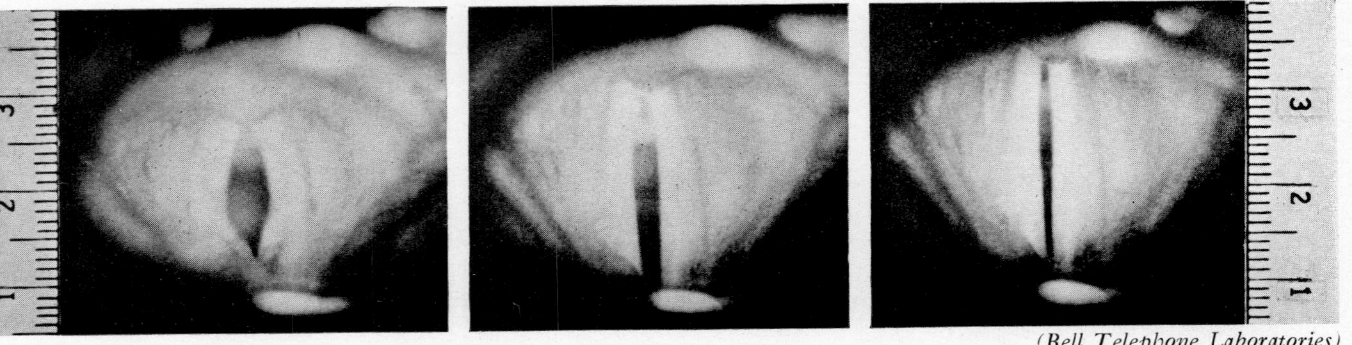

(Bell Telephone Laboratories)

PLATE II. Elongation of Vocal Cords

The photographs represent three stages of stretching of the vocal cords in singing (left to right) a B, b and e^1. The marginal scales do not indicate actual size in inches; they are added to permit comparison of length of vocal cords at various pitches.

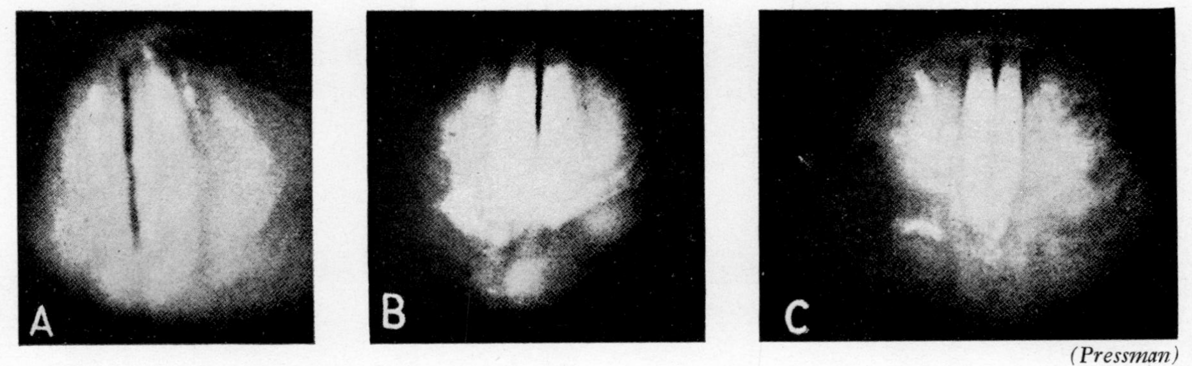

(Pressman)

PLATE III. Vocal Cords in High Tones

Three stages of the damping mechanism of the vocal cords. With increasing pitch the vocal cords become more approximated in the posterior part until, in the highest falsetto, only a small anterior segment is left free to vibrate.

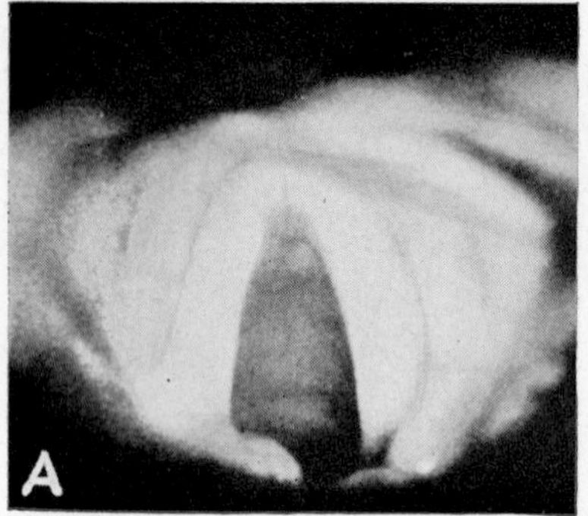

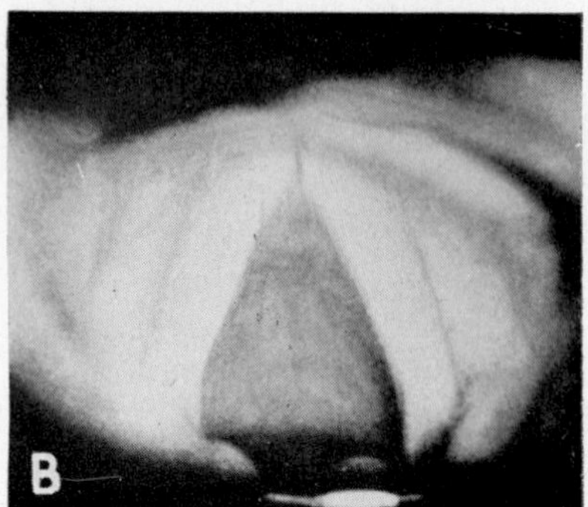

PLATE IV. Vocal Cords in Breathing

A. Position of cords in quiet respiration
B. Breathing in moderate effort
C. Breathing in extreme exertion

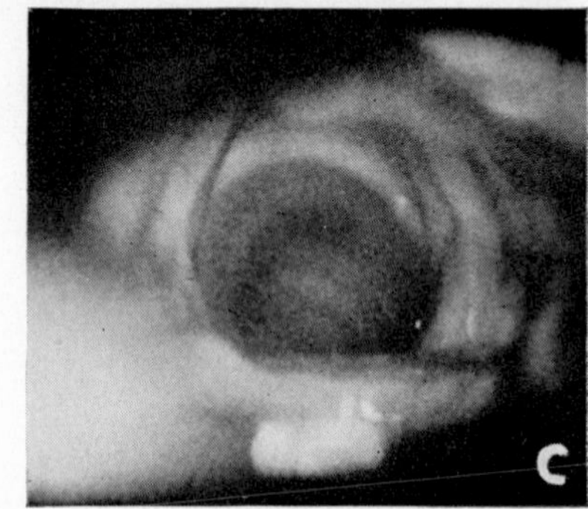

(Bell Telephone Laboratories)

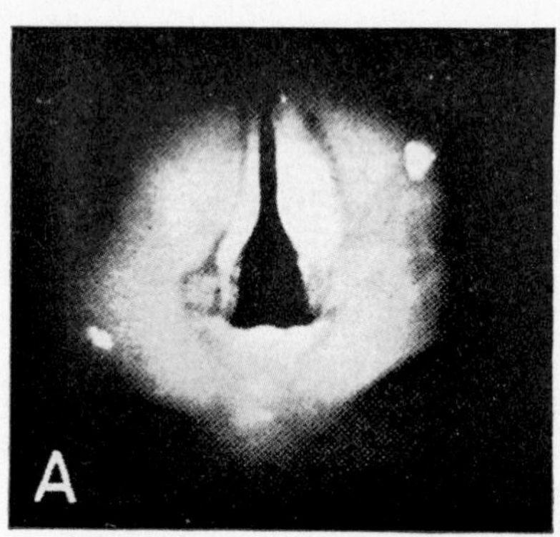

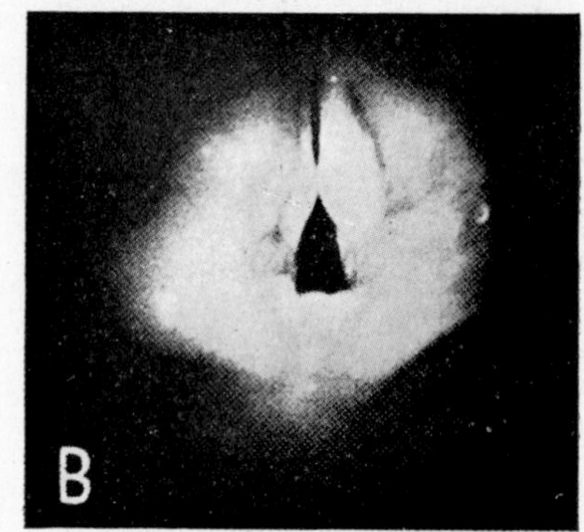

(Pressman)

PLATE V. Vocal Cords in Whispering

A. Represents a low-pitched whisper without effort
B. A more forceful whisper at higher pitch

The mouth and the throat are moistened by *saliva*, the product of large glands in the the cheeks (parotid glands) and in the floor of the mouth (submaxillary and sublingual glands). When we eat, the mechanical effect of chewing stimulates and increases flow of saliva. In addition, purely nervous impulses control the production of saliva and the action of the mucous glands. The sight of appetizing food, even the thought of it, makes our mouth water.

On the other hand apprehension and anxiety inhibit the glands. The result is the dry mouth, tongue and throat, a well-known experience with public speakers, actors and singers before an appearance. When the first applause has restored the confidence, opposing impulses bring the normal flow of saliva and mucous back within a few minutes.

We all know the nose as the seat of the sense of smell but even more important is its function as a magnificent air-conditioning unit of great simplicity. In the very short time it takes for the air to travel from the nostrils to the throat it is warmed to body temperature, humidified to a level of comfort for the mucous membranes and cleaned. The folded surface of the lateral wall of the nose provides a maximum of contact with the air which is further increased by the curved pathway the air takes—up to the roof of the nasal cavity and down to the throat.

The size of the turbinates can be increased by filling their vessels with blood, adapting the nose to changes of temperature and dryness and following all kinds of nervous and even emotional impulses. We shall encounter this important fact frequently later on.

We have to tell you much less about the mouth because there you are on familiar ground. Let us just mention a few facts that have bearing on voice and speech. The *tongue* is a much larger organ than we usually assume. The little boy who sticks out his tongue in defiance as widely as he can brings only the anterior part of it into the open. As you see in Fig. 1

the tongue forms a large muscular mass of criss-crossing muscle fibers which give the tongue its extraordinary flexibility and motility. We do not want to hurt your feelings when we say that a completely dissected human tongue does not differ much in size and shape from a small calf's tongue you can see in a butcher store.

The soft *palate* with the attachment of the uvula serves as a curtain which can be raised or lowered by muscular action. If we breathe through the nose it hangs down in relaxation and permits the passage of air into the throat. If we swallow it is raised against the throat, thereby sealing off the nasal cavity against penetration of food. The strong muscles of the throat do the rest and the food is pressed downward into the gullet or *esophagus*.

Again, speech has come to the mouth as a late achievement, while chewing of the food is the common function of the mouth in many animals and men—a fact we should remember for later discussions.

We have to mention one more set of structures in the mouth which take no part in eating, breathing or speaking but are important to health because of their nuisance value: tonsils and adenoids.

Together they form a ring of so-called lymphatic tissue around the throat. The *adenoids* as you can see in Fig. 2 form a small cushion at the roof of the throat behind the soft palate. Normally, they are present in childhood and disappear near puberty. If enlarged they block the passage of air from the nose leaving the mouth as the only free avenue. The *tonsils*, best known structures of the group, lie on both sides of the tongue between folds of mucous membrane in which muscles run up to the soft palate. Similar tissue is found at the base of the tongue, arranged in two small lumps that meet in the mid-line. If infected, it can form larger masses which are called *lingual tonsils* (*lingua* being the Latin name of the tongue and the root of the adjective linguistic). Such large

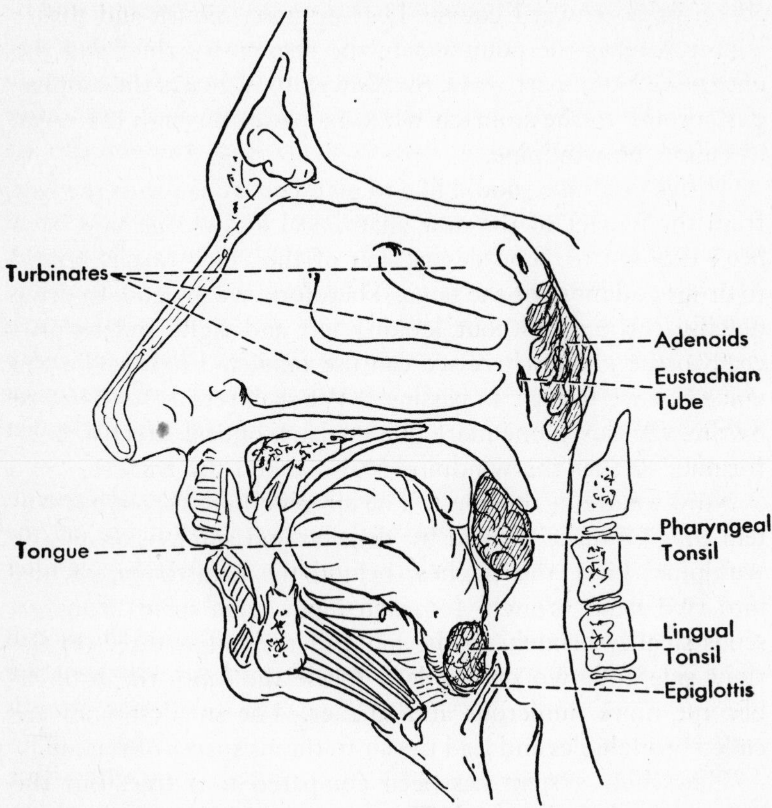

FIG. 2. The Tonsillar Ring

The cross section is the same as in Fig. 1 except that the tongue has been pushed aside. The adenoids, pharyngeal and lingual tonsils are visible.

lingual tonsils can form, as we shall see, a bottleneck which prevents the free development of the voice.

Behind the wall of the throat run a number of strong muscles. Aside from their action in swallowing they are able to change the form of the throat and thus modify the sound of the voice.

As you might remember we meant to trace the pathway of

air on its downward course. Leaving nose, mouth and throat it now reaches the point where the respiratory tract and the digestive system part ways. Swallowed food enters the esophagus enroute to the stomach while air passes through the voice box into the windpipe.

At this point we should like to give you a chance to recover from the impact of the new anatomical knowledge you have been exposed to. The description of the voice box is bound to bring you more of the same. Therefore, we propose to drive quickly through without looking left and right and to proceed to the chest where we can use familiar English. To the voice box we just say in passing: "We shall return" and notice on the way down one more bilingual anatomical street sign informing us that the windpipe is also called the *trachea.*

Now we are in the chest. The air gets there through a system of pipe lines, formed by division and subdivision of the windpipe. First, the trachea, behind the breastbone, divides into two main bronchi for each lung. Each main bronchus sends smaller bronchi to the lobes of the lungs, three on the right side and two on the left. Inside the lobes the bronchi become more numerous and smaller. The smallest ones are called bronchioles and lead the air to the air spaces of the lungs.

The whole system has been compared to a tree. But the bronchial tree is inverted. The windpipe, the trunk, is above the branches of the bronchi and bronchioles which hang down. To keep the windpipe and the bronchi from collapsing when air is sucked into the lungs the walls of these pipe lines are fortified by rings of elastic cartilage.

The *lungs* fill the whole chest with the exception of a space in the middle where we find the heart, the esophagus, large blood vessels and nerves. The chest itself is a cage formed by the ribs, the spine and the breastbone.

Lungs and heart both rest on the *diaphragm.* It got its name from the Greek word for partition and that's what it is. The diaphragm separates the cavities of the chest and the abdomen.

Since we shall have to talk a great deal about the function of the diaphragm we better describe it to you in more detail.

The diaphragm is a large muscle. Almost all the other muscles connect two points of the skeleton. By their contraction they shorten the distance between these points thereby changing the position of the bones they are attached to. The muscle fibers of the diaphragm originate from the lower ribs, the breastbone and the spine but they converge like the spokes of a wheel at the center which consists of tough tendinous tissue. In relaxed position the diaphragm is dome-shaped. When the muscle fibers contract the dome is flattened and the center moves *down*. Please keep this fact in mind. We shall need it in the next chapter when we discuss the mechanism of breathing.

The lungs are covered by a protective layer of fibrous tissue, the *pleura*. A second sheet of pleura lines the inside of the chest. Both layers are connected and form the pleural sack which contains a lubricating substance to facilitate the movements of the lungs. There is no air in the pleural sack which acts like a large suction cup that fixes the surface of the lungs to the chest wall. When the chest expands—by the elevation of the ribs—the lungs are unfolded and filled with air.

The cage of the chest is formed by the twelve pairs of *ribs*. They are flat bones, bent in a curvature and relatively thin, which exposes them to fractures when a severer force hits the chest. They are connected in the rear to the bones of the spine by joints with a limited freedom of motion. The first seven ribs are attached to the breastbone, the next three to the higher ribs by bands of elastic cartilage which give the chest a springy motility. The two lowest ribs are short and do not reach the breastbone. They do not take part in the movements of the chest.

Muscles between the ribs and others that are attached to the outside of the chest move the ribs up and down. The joints in the rear give leverage to the ribs which can be raised to a more horizontal position. This leads to a deepening of the chest and,—in the lower half—to a sideward expansion. In this position which is fullest in the extreme of deep inspiration the chest has reached its greatest capacity. Moving the ribs downward contracts the chest in all dimensions, thus squeezing the air out of the lungs. We shall discuss this mechanism in more detail in the next chapter.

Leaving the air spaces of the lungs on expiration, the air passes through the bronchioles, smaller and larger bronchi and finally the windpipe until it reaches the voice box which we have, so far, neglected.

By now, we better give the voice box its proper name, the *larynx*. All the medical terms for the voice box and its details are of Greek origin, proof of the interest this organ has attracted since the times of antiquity. The Greek physician Galen who lived in the second century has described and named the larger cartilages of the larynx. The first drawings of the cartilages, the vocal cords and of the whole larynx in profile were made in 1490 by Leonardo da Vinci whose studies of the vocal organs Dr. Panconcelli-Calzia has lately compiled and reproduced in a beautiful volume. In the sixteenth century, Vesalius of Padua made complete dissections of the larynx that are hardly surpassed today in accuracy and detail.

The first important fact that all anatomists have noticed about the larynx is the ingenious method of suspension which anticipates the use of springs in modern technical design. Above, from the jaw and the base of the skull and below, from breastbone and collarbone, muscles reach out to provide elastic suspension for the larynx and the windpipe on the top of which the voice box rides.

This arrangement permits not only free movements of the larynx with the head and neck but gives protection to the larynx against impact of any force that hits the neck.

Above the larynx the muscles that hold it are stabilized by the insertion of a thin bone of horseshoe form (with the prongs pointing to the rear in a horizontal plane). You can feel this *hyoid bone* if you take the region slightly above your voice box between thumb and index finger.

Added protection is given to the voice box by the fact that it is made up of highly elastic cartilage. A fracture of the larynx is a severe and sometimes fatal accident. Free suspension and elasticity make it a rather rare event.

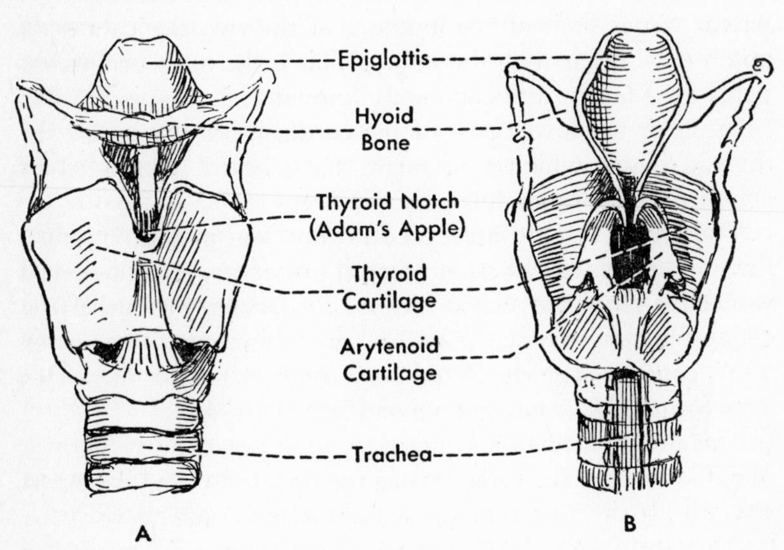

FIG. 3. The Larynx

A. Front view B. Rear view

The larynx consists of nine cartilages of which we intend to bother you only with five. The remaining four are tiny, unimportant and belong to the large group of insignificant detail that haunts the nights of medical students before anatomy tests.

One cartilage belongs to the tongue almost as much as to the larynx. It is called *epiglottis* and has the shape of a teaspoon with the handle sawed off (Fig. 3). You find it on the cross section of Fig. 1 too, if you look at the base of the tongue.

When we swallow, the epiglottis tilts backward until it lies like a lid over the entrance of the larynx. The food then glides over it into the esophagus.

The "box" of the larynx is made up of two larger cartilages. The bigger one of the two consists of two wings which meet in front at a steep angle. Looking like an antique soldier's shield it carries the Greek name for "shield like," *thyroid cartilage.* At the upper limit of the juncture of the two shields a deep notch can be felt with the finger. This is the most prominent part of the larynx and commonly known as the Adam's apple. In front of the lower part of the cartilage lies the important thyroid gland which you might have heard mentioned in connection with glandular disturbances.

The wings as they are called do not join in the rear thus leaving open space where no special protection is needed, and where the esophagus begins behind the larynx. From the free ends of the wings two pairs of horns stick out. The upper horns connect with the hyoid bone through a band, the lower ones form a joint with the second large cartilage.

This one looks like a signet ring, with the stone facing the rear. Galen used the Greek word for ring and called it *cricoid cartilage.* It sits on top of the windpipe and connects with the thyroid cartilage by the joint we just mentioned. This makes a tilting motion of the thyroid against the cricoid cartilage possible which, as we shall see, is of importance in varying the tension of the vocal cords.

In the rear of the cricoid, on the upper rim of the "signet stone," ride two small cartilages of the shape of a pyramid with a triangular base and a tip that is slightly bent. This gives them the appearance of a pitcher and bestowed on them the tongue-twisting name of *arytenoid cartilages.* (Again we apologize in the name of the medical profession for all these unwieldy names. They are two thousand years old and must have given the same disgust you probably feel to countless generations of students.)

The joints that connect the arytenoids with the cricoid cartilage make two kinds of movement possible. The little pyramids can approach each other or become separated, and they can turn around an axis from the tip to the middle of the base.

This is of greatest importance because attached to the anterior corners of the pyramids that face each other are the *vocal cords.* All the structures we have mentioned so far have just one purpose: to house, protect, move and tense the vocal cords. Since in this book we shall speak about the vocal cords more than about any other organ they deserve a special place in our description.

It is strange to see how long the function of the vocal cords was overlooked. Even Leonardo da Vinci with his incredibly sharp eyes for detail hardly marked the cords in his drawing and believed that the voice was created in the windpipe. In 1741, Antoine Ferrein in Paris was the first scientist to understand these neglected structures as vibrating strings and called them *cordes vocales.*

The vocal cords are attached in front to the inside of the thyroid cartilage where the two wings meet. This is the fixed point where the cords always touch each other. In the rear, as we just mentioned, they are connected with the anterior corner of the arytenoids. There, they can be opened and closed, lying together on closing and forming a triangular chink on opening. This space between the opened cords is called the *glottis.*

Since this is a fundamental point in our discussions we should like to make absolutely sure that we understand each other. For a simple demonstration we have to ask you to get up from your chair (you might welcome anyhow the opportunity to stretch your legs after this onslaught of necessary but tedious detail). Stand with your feet together. They represent the vocal cords. Where the tips of your shoes are is the firm connection of the cords with the thyroid cartilage, while the heels mark the attachment of the cords to the arytenoids. Then, spread your feet at the heels, leaving the tips of your shoes together and you have the true position of the vocal cords inside the larynx: horizontal, inseparable in front, but able to spread wide in the rear.

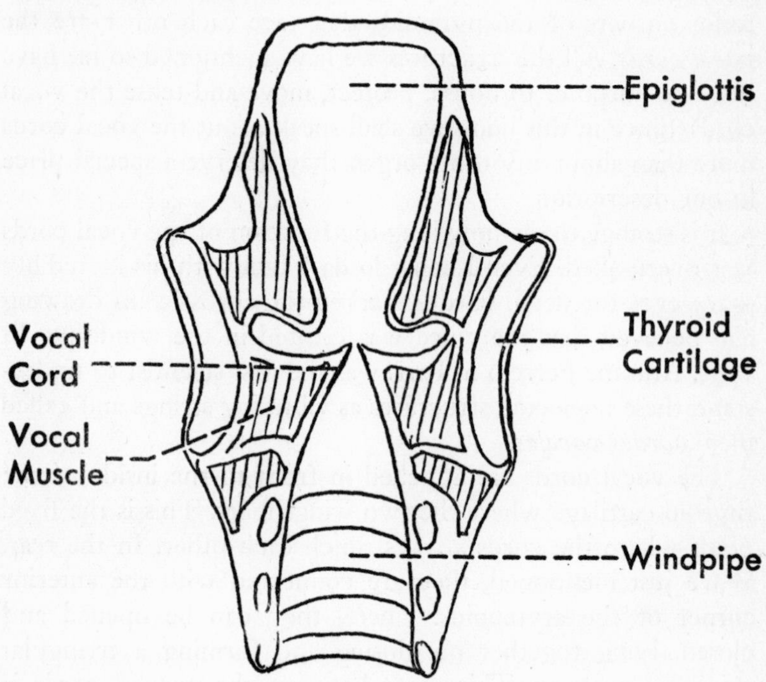

FIG. 4. Cross Section of the Larynx

On the view of the larynx you see in Fig. 4 the shape of the cords becomes clearer. They are not flat bands but rather heavy and triangular on cross section. While the upper surface is flat in the horizontal, the lower surface slants at an angle that makes the cords thinnest at the free edges and heaviest on the outside. This slant helps to slide the air in singing and speaking against the point of contact of the cords.

It is, by the way, one of the reasons why we can sing only on exhalation. Some of the birds who have special organs, called syringes, deep down in the windpipe can sing for minutes, on inhaling as well as on expiration.

The upper surface and the free margins which have to withstand a lot of force are covered with a tough kind of cells, somewhat similar to the top layer of our skin, while the rest of the larynx is lined with the usual mucous membrane. This accounts for the white appearance of the cords when seen from above as on examination with the laryngeal mirror.

At this point we should like to mention that not all otherwise normal cords are white. We see all nuances of pinkish-gray, particularly in deep voices. What is already a symptom of laryngitis for one speaker or singer may be the normal appearance for others and just the result of years of hard work like the calluses on the hands of a working man.

All normal cords have a smooth, glistening surface, due to a thin layer of mucus that covers them. Above the cords as you see in Fig. 4 are folds of mucous membrane, called the *false cords*. They have no special significance under normal conditions.

It remains only to tell you something about the *muscles* which move and tense the vocal cords. There is not much sense in bothering you with the rather complicated names of these muscles. Except for laryngologists few doctors would be able to identify the function of such tongue twisters as for instance the "thyroarytenoid muscle."

Just look at a few drawings in Fig. 5 which explain the opening and closing of the glottis in a schematical way. You see the cords the way they are visible from above. The pyramids of the arytenoid cartilages appear as little triangles, to the anterior corner of which the posterior ends of the vocal cords are attached. The frontal ends of the cords—above in the figures—are fixed inside of the thyroid cartilages.

Two pairs of tiny muscles go from the cricoid cartilage to

the outer angles of the pyramids. If the posterior pair contracts they pull in the direction of the arrows in A. The pyramids are turned outward and with it the vocal cords. They open wide leaving the triangular chink of the glottis between them. This is the position they assume when we breathe.

If the lateral pair of muscles contract the arytenoids are turned inward (B) and the vocal cords are brought together, but in the rear an opening remains between the cartilages.

To close the last gap muscle fibers which run from one arytenoid to the other one contract, thus pulling them together (C). The closure of the cords is finished. This is the position for the production of voice.

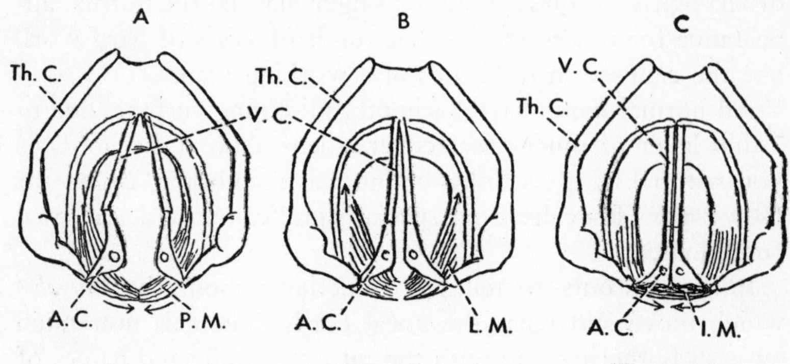

(Pressman)

FIG. 5. Opening and Closing of the Vocal Cords

Th.C.—thyroid cartilage. A.C.—arytenoid cartilages. V.C.—vocal cords.

In A the cords are opened by the action of the posterior muscles (P.M.).

In B the cords are closed by the action of the lateral muscle (L.M.), but a chink remains open in the posterior part.

The closing is completed (C) by the action of the interarytenoid muscle (I.M.).

But they cannot yet vibrate without being tensed. This is achieved by creating tension within and from without.

Through the whole length of each vocal cord runs a muscle. In Fig. 4 you see it in cross section. Contraction of this muscle makes the cords thicker, shorter and more tense.

The tensing from without is produced by an ingenious mechanism. As you may remember the thyroid cartilage can be tilted against the cricoid. This movement, which is achieved by another muscle, lengthens the distance between the two points of attachment of the vocal cords. Result: the cords are stretched, becoming longer, thinner and more tense.

Both mechanisms, increase of the inner tension of the cords and stretching by outside pull, combine to produce any desired degree of tension, length and thickness of the vocal cords.

You can visualize this interplay of forces by using one of the flat rubber bands that are used to hold small parcels. If you take one loop in one hand so that the two sections of the band are parallel and approximated, and pull the other end you will observe the thinning of the bands while you feel the increased inner tension of the stretched bands.

This finishes our excursion into the anatomy of the vocal organs. Do not worry if some of the many new names and terms have already escaped your memory. You will later on see that we did not mention a single structure which will not have some significance in our coming discussions. And then, you can always refresh your memory by looking back at the illustrations of this chapter.

Having understood the structures of the larynx we can now proceed in the next chapter to the study of the mechanism of voice production.

III. *Queen of the Instruments*

The stage is set for the great aria of "Lenore" in Beethoven's *Fidelio*. A stormy recitative paints the uproar of the elements with strings and woodwinds. Three horns, one after the other one, introduce a moving phrase in the radiant yet mellow harmonies of E-major.

But then, the voice emerges again, the voice of a woman who trembles for her captive husband, and suddenly all the instruments of the orchestra pale beside the flexibility, the grandeur and the richness of this singular instrument. It sings of fear, of despair and of prayerful hope until it finally erupts into the quickened pulses of courage and determination. One cannot hear this masterpiece of musical creation interpreted by a great singer without being touched to tears.

It is not a powerful instrument, this human voice, nor a technically perfect one. A trumpet can blow louder, a violin play faster, an oboe spin longer melodies. Still, it is unsurpassed in expressivity, depth and soulfulness of tone, truly the queen of instruments.

It is not the property of the singer alone. It colors every word we say with emotional undertones, with pathos or humble resignation, with energy or deadly fear, with persuasiveness or deceit.

We use this instrument daily, still know very little about it. This chapter intends to introduce you to the mechanics of the voice. We are still far away from having all the answers about the function and the acoustics of the voice. Many details are still hotly argued about. But we can, at least, explain satisfactorily the basic facts of voice production in somewhat simplified terms.

Whether we use the voice in speaking or singing we produce—in acoustical terms—vibrations of air. Every audible sound consists of such vibrations, rhythmical ones in music, irregular ones in noise. To leave the latter out for the time being, we can say that to every musical note corresponds a rhythmical vibration of air of a certain number per second, called *frequency*. From the point of origin the *waves* of sound spread in all directions, weakening in the square of distance until they die away. The greater the motion of vibrating air the greater the *amplitude* or intensity of the sound.

Outside of experimental setups hardly any pure tones are produced in nature. Any sound that emanates from an instrument or from the voice consists of a basic tone, the *fundamental* and a number of related *overtones* or *partials*, usually multiples of the basic frequency. The mixture of the fundamental with partials of varying strength accounts for the color or quality which distinguishes for our ear the same note if played by a violin or an oboe, by a flute or a clarinet, or if sung by a soprano or an alto.

Every note of our harmonic system has a certain frequency or *pitch*. The intervals we use in all kinds of musical compositions can be expressed in relations of frequencies. The higher note of an octave has twice the number of vibrations as the lower one. The major triad—the basis of our musical system—has frequency values of 4:5:6. The following table gives the frequency relations of some intervals:

Unison	1:1	Fourth	4:3
Major third	5:4	Fifth	3:2
Minor third	6:5	Octave	2:1

Instruments can be classified according to the mechanics they employ in creating vibrations of air. We can best understand the mechanism of the human voice if we compare it to the major instrumental groups of the orchestra.

Woodwinds and brass instruments are both, acoustically speaking, *pipes*. A column of air, enclosed in a wooden or metal pipe, is made to vibrate.

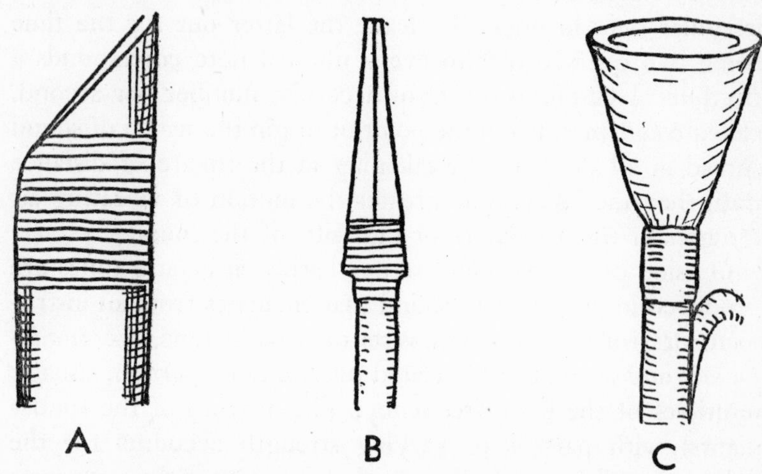

FIG. 6. Mouthpieces of Musical Instruments
A. Clarinet B. Oboe C. Trumpet

In the *woodwinds*, with the exception of the flute, this is achieved by the action of *reeds*. Flat pieces of thin slices of cane are mounted on a mouthpiece. When blown against, they begin to vibrate, opening and closing the entrance of the mouthpiece. The steady stream of air is rhythmically interrupted, and the resulting vibration of air is transmitted to the air in the wooden body of the instrument. While the clarinet employs a single reed, the oboe and the bassoon have mouthpieces with two reeds in close contact (see Fig. 6). In the opening phase they swing away from each other, separated by the pressure of air and return again to the closed position by their elasticity. The vibration of the vocal cords has been compared to this double-reed action.

But the principle of action of the *brass instruments* gives an even better illustration. Here, the lips of the player are the source of air vibration. Pressed under tension into the funnel-shaped mouthpiece, they open and close to the blowing stream of air in quick succession. The tense but rounded margins of the lips act like vibrating cushions which have given to this type of instrument the acoustic name of *cushion pipes*.

The vocal cords are such cushion pipes. Closed and tensed, they resist the pressure of air in the trachea until they are blown apart. A puff of air escapes and lowers the air pressure below. The temporary decrease of pressure permits the closure of the cords by their inner tension and elasticity. This interplay of forces achieves a fast rhythmical change of opening and closing, thus transforming the steady stream of air into rhythmical vibrations. The tone is born.

In most pipe instruments the *pitch* of the sound they produce depends on the length of the vibrating air column. The shorter the column the higher the pitch. Through a system of keys or valves which open holes to the escape of air the length of the pipe can be varied and a series of different tones produced.

The human voice employs a different principle to achieve changes in pitch: the increase or decrease of the tension of the vocal cords. We find the same principle used in all *string instruments*. A violin, for instance, is tuned to the desired pitch by turning the pegs which hold the strings, thereby changing the tension. The higher the tension the faster the vibrations and the higher the produced note. The fingering in playing the string instruments has the same effect. By shortening the vibrating part of the string it thus increases the tension and raises the pitch.

Increase or decrease of the tension of the vocal cords is

achieved by the muscular mechanism we discussed in the last chapter. If we want to sing a higher note after a lower one we increase the tension of the cords and thus make them vibrate at a faster rate.

If you tie a piece of string at one end and pull the other end hard you can produce a whole series of sounds by plucking the string at different degrees of tension.

The intensity or *loudness* of a given note depends on the degree of air pressure from below. The harder we blow against the cords the wider the vibrating excursions of the cords and the louder the sound our voice produces.

Actually, increase in air pressure raises the pitch to a certain degree but a fine adjustment of the tensing muscles of the cords compensates for this effect. For our purposes we can stick to our definition: increased tension of the cords raises the pitch, increased pressure of air fortifies the intensity of the sound.

The frequency of a given tone determines the speed with which the cords vibrate. The deepest notes of a basso require around 60 vibrations of the cords per second. For the a^1 on the second space of our usual treble clef—the so-called chamber A—440 vibrations are necessary. But for the high c^3 of a soprano the vocal cords have to open and close at the incredible speed of 1,046 per second.

Observations with the high-speed camera—which we shall discuss in Chapter IX—have taught us a great deal about the vibrations of the cords. They do not close or open in a straight line but in a rather undulating fashion. In slow motion it looks as if a blanket is shaken in waves. This means that at no time in singing is the whole length of the cords completely closed.

There exists a fundamental difference in the type of vibration at low and high tones. In producing low notes the cords swing wide with a movement that envelops the whole mass of the cords. The higher the note the more limited becomes the vibration to the free borders of the cords. Finally, in the highest notes the cords remain in close contact in the posterior part, leaving only the anterior half or third free to vibrate. In this stage the cords are tense, show no motion in the rear and vibrate in the frontal part only at the sharpened inner margins.

For a better visualization of the motion of the cords you should now turn to Plates I-V. They show a number of rather unusual photographs taken under different conditions of vocal use.

Plate I shows a set of photographs of the cords during one full cycle of opening and closing in singing. They are single exposures which were taken out of a film that was obtained with the high-speed camera of the Bell Telephone Laboratories. Since the singer during this shot produced a note of about 260 vibrations the set of the six photographs covers the time of 1/260 second.

Plate II (from the same film) shows the cords of a baritone singing three different notes. The second one is one octave higher than the first, the third one one-fifth higher than the second. The higher the note the thinner and longer the cords become by the stretching pull, as you can see with the help of the measuring scales at the sides of the photos.

Plate III shows the position of the cords in singing high notes. At the beginning of the head register (A) the cords are stretched but still vibrate at full length. Higher up (B) the cords are approximated (damped) at the posterior half, leaving the anterior half free to vibrate. In falsetto (C) the cords are damped in the two posterior thirds; only a small triangular chink is open in the anterior third where the sharpened margins vibrate.

Plate IV illustrates the different degrees of cord opening in breathing, from quiet respiration (A), to moderate work (B), such as walking on the street, and to breathing in extreme exertion (C) with wide open cords, between which the upper rings of the windpipe can be seen.

We should like to mention here the position of the cords in *whispering* because of its great practical importance. Plate V shows the cords both in toneless (A) and in more forceful "stage" whisper (B). You see that in both instances the cords are approaching each other, in the forceful whisper to the point of contact. In both conditions they vibrate. Therefore, whispering is *no* rest for the vocal cords. If voice rest is needed for a patient, whispering should be forbidden as well as speaking.

So far, we have discussed only the vocal cords as the source of sound. If we heard only the sounds the cords produce we would perceive a weak tinny voice, hardly audible at more than a few feet distance. The same applies to most musical instruments. The strings of a violin, for instance, would produce only a very weak sound without the help of the resonating body of the instrument.

By *resonance* we describe any process by which the energy of a musical sound is augmented. The weak vibrations of the strings of the violin are taken over and reinforced by the vibrations of the wooden body of the instrument which, in turn, incites the air inside the body to strong vibrations, all resulting in a tone of great intensity. The body is the resonator of the violin.

Such resonators can be selective: sharply attuned to one single frequency, such as the pipes of an organ. Or they can be broad resonators which amplify a wide range of sounds. The horn of a loudspeaker, the bell of the brass instruments, the sounding board of a piano are such broad resonators.

The resonator of the human voice is unique because its shape can be partly altered. Of the organs which enclose the air column above the vocal cords only the nose is a rigid structure. The shape of the throat and, more so, of the mouth, tongue and lips can be changed by muscular action. As we shall see, speech is made possible by changes of the resonating cavities, and the quality of musical sound in singing can be considerably altered by conscious or subconscious modifications of the resonators.

The human resonator is prevalently of the broad type. Hard and rigid resonators have a more selective effect than those with softer surfaces that give a more general reinforcement of sounds. This result is based on the filtering out of overtones by absorption, the so-called damping effect. Selective resonance produces more powerful tones, but the soft and changeable walls of the human resonator permit the production of a wide range of usable sounds.

Resonance is not limited to the air spaces above the vocal cords. To a certain extent the air in the windpipe and bronchi takes part in the amplification of sound, particularly in the deep tones up to frequencies of 250. While speaking with our deepest voice or singing in the low range we can feel the resonating vibrations in our chest.

At this point we should like to say a word about *vibrations* as body sensations. Many speakers when addressing large crowds in a strong voice and most singers when singing loud can feel all kinds of vibrations in the palate, the nose, the forehead and in other places. These sensations have led many teachers to the false concept that sound could be "directed" selectively to such parts of the body. From one individual to another one, the body sensations vary greatly; they have no significance for the right or wrong use of the voice and are no key to the improvement of singing or speaking techniques.

Whether we speak or sing, we always use the vocal organs as a unit. The physicists call it a *coupled system.* That means that its sound-producing parts, the vocal cords with the air columns above and below, act together, one influencing, reinforcing and stimulating the vibrations of the other. Any teaching theory that picks out a single sensation or movement as a guide to perfection leaves the firm basis of scientific fact.

So far, we have discussed the vocal cords which are the source of voice sounds and the resonating cavities which step

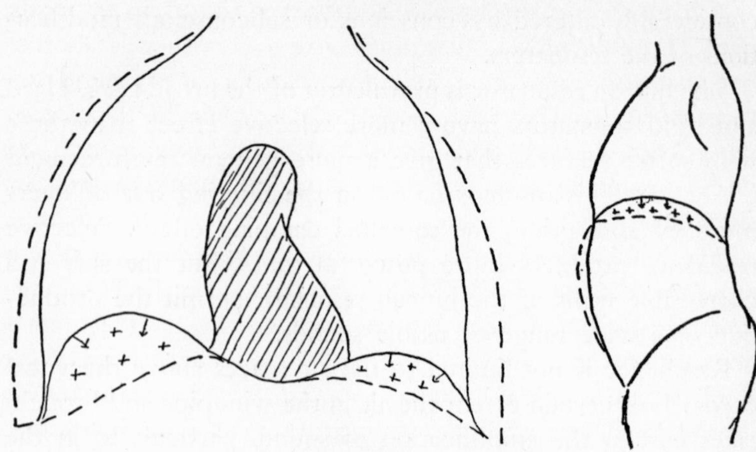

Fig. 7. The Mechanics of Breathing

A. Chest breathing. In deep expiration (solid lines) the diaphragm goes up and the chest contracts. In deep inspiration (broken lines) the chest expands and the diaphragm flattens by contraction; the space gained by the descent of the diaphragm is marked by + signs. The shaded area represents the heart.

B. Abdominal breathing. In deep expiration the abdominal wall is contracted while the diaphragm relaxes (goes up). In deep inspiration (broken lines) the abdominal wall relaxes (protrudes) while the diaphragm contracts (flattens).

up the volume of sound to its full dynamic possibilities. It remains to consider the bellows which provide the air pressure and drives the vocal cords to vibration.

In the last chapter we have already described the mechanism of the *chest* in *breathing*, based on the raising and lowering of the ribs. This breathing by expansion and contraction of the chest is supplemented by *abdominal breathing*. You will remember that we stressed the fact that the dome-shaped diaphragm flattens and descends on contraction during deep inspiration (Fig. 7A).

All muscles of the human body are arranged in opposing pairs. To each muscle or muscle group corresponds another one that acts as its antagonist. For instance, if we bend our forearm we contract the biceps muscle while its antagonist, the triceps, relaxes. This muscle, in turn, takes over if we wish to extend the arm. Then, the triceps contracts and the antagonist, the biceps, relaxes.

The antagonists of the diaphragm are the muscles which tense the abdominal wall (belly and flanks). In deep inspiration the diaphragm contracts and moves down. This exerts pressure on the organs which fill the abdominal cavity, liver, stomach, intestines and others. To escape the downward pressure from above they begin to protrude. This is made possible by the relaxation of the abdominal muscles. The result of this mechanism is: more air space in the chest because of the flattening of the diaphragm, expansion of the belly to accommodate the protruding abdominal organs (Fig. 7B).

Now, let us consider what happens in deep expiration, for instance, while we speak or sing. The diaphragm relaxes and the abdominal muscles contract. The abdominal organs are compressed by the contracting muscles. To escape this pressure they move inward and upward, pushing the relaxing diaphragm into the chest, thus squeezing air out of the lungs. At the end of a deep expiration the wall of abdomen and flanks is pulled in, the relaxed diaphragm has risen until it has assumed its dome shape (Fig. 7B).

This interplay of forces, if done well, goes very smoothly; contraction and relaxation are perfected in slow transitions. But one fact is clear from this explanation: in abdominal inspiration the driving force is the diaphragm while the expiration is controlled by the abdominal muscles. The term *diaphragmatical control* which has become such a favorite with teachers of singing and speaking is somewhat misleading. During expiration, when we create air pressure to make the vocal cords vibrate, it is the abdominal muscles that do the real work.

True, a smooth control of expiration depends to a certain degree on the slow relaxation of the diaphragm. But another factor prevents a conscious control of the diaphragm. Of all the muscles of the human body the diaphragm is the only one without a sense of position. Even with closed eyes we are always aware of the position of all parts of our body.

In breathing, we can feel the action of all parts involved. We are aware of the expansion or contraction of our chest. We can feel the contraction or the bulging of our belly and our flanks. But we cannot become aware of the position of our diaphragm in breathing. For this reason it would be better to speak of *abdominal control*, but diaphragmatical control has become such a favorite with the singing profession that the term will stay, regardless of the functional facts. Not much harm will be done as long as you are fully aware of the antagonistic interplay of both muscle groups.

We all use chest and abdominal breathing together. As a rule chest breathing is more pronounced in women and abdominal breathing in men. The goal of a proper training of the speaking and singing voice is to strengthen the less developed mechanism and to blend both into one single smoothly functioning unit. There is no prescription for ideal breathing that fits everybody. It is the task of the good teacher to find out which form of breathing gives the best results in an individual student.

The trouble with too many systems of vocal instruction is that they try to make everybody conform to a rigid set of motions and actions. Some of the best singers have used highly irregular positions and movements of their vocal organs. And the brilliant result that a system has achieved with one student does not prove that it will be successful with others. The best teacher is the one who is able to develop the possibilities of each student by flexible methods and techniques.

In quiet breathing the expiration takes about one half more time than the inspiration. This ratio is changed in speaking or singing when the expiration becomes prolonged enough to permit the speaking of whole sentences or the singing of complete musical phrases in one breath. Nose breathing, which permits the intake of air at a slower rate only, becomes insufficient for the needs of speedy inspiration in speaking and singing—as it does in strenuous exercise—and then we switch to mouth breathing.

The beneficial effect of nose breathing is still preserved because even the busiest speaker or singer keeps his mouth closed for the greater part of the day. Aside from the air-conditioning function of the nose, nasal breathing is of great importance to the strengthening of the voice. If you breathe first through mouth and then through the nose you will notice the resistance that the narrower pathway of the nose offers to breathing. This helps to develop the muscles which are involved both in inspiration and expiration, particularly in the younger individual.

Now, we can bring the whole picture into focus. We have discussed the mechanism of breathing which provides air pressure below the vocal cords. The cords which are closed and tensed at the beginning of phonation are blown apart by the mounting air pressure in the trachea and then made to vibrate by the interplay of pressure from below and elastic resistance in the cords. The resulting vibration creates a sound which is amplified in the resonating cavities. Pitch depends on the frequency of vibration of the cords, volume of sound on the pressure of air against the cords.

We still shall have to discuss a number of details which are important for the understanding of artistic singing. But before doing so we should like to study first the mechanics of speech, the characteristics of the speaking voice and the requirements for professional speech. We shall use the next two chapters for this purpose. We shall then return to the singing voice in Chapter VI which, to the singer, will be the continuation of this one.

Before we can close this chapter we have to touch on one more subject: functions of the larynx aside from the production of voice.

We started our anatomical description with the remark that the larynx appears first in the amphibians as a safety valve against penetration of water into the newly developed lungs. With the economy that is so characteristic of the evolution in nature this valve was maintained in the mammals but adapted to new functions. They have to do with the building up of air pressure in the chest by tight closure of the cords during expiration.

It began when some animals developed the ability to do heavy work with their forelimbs while squatting on their haunches. They learned to get added strength for lifting heavy objects by suddenly closing the cords and pressing air against them. This transforms the chest into a rigid cage which gives the muscles of the forelimb that are attached to it greater power and a firmer grip.

Man who has transformed his forelimbs into the adaptable and versatile tools of the arms uses this technique constantly. If we want to lift a heavy crate we first close our vocal cords tightly, build up air pressure by contraction of the chest and abdominal muscles and then use the muscles of the arms. The work done we release the air with an audible rush and resume normal breathing.

Patients who have lost the ability to close the cords or who have to wear a cannula in the trachea after an operation are severely handicapped for heavy work.

We might mention here that the evolution from the animal who walks on four legs to man's erect posture has been paid for by choking up his airways. In assuming this posture the pathway of air in the throat has become bent at a sharp angle. When running fast we assume instinctively the animal position of the head by thrusting our chin forward and upward, thus straightening out the intake of air for greater efficiency.

Another use of the larynx as a valve is made in *coughing* when we use the sudden release of pressure behind the closed cords to eject mucus from trachea and bronchi with the rush of escaping air.

One more use of the pressure-valve mechanism is made in bowel *movements* when the compressed air in the chest forces the diaphragm down, thus providing pressure on the intestines in teamwork with the contracting abdominal muscles.

All in all, it is the story of the versatility of nature we have followed in the last two chapters. Dr. V. E. Negus, a famous English throat specialist, has written a fascinating study of the evolutionary history of the larynx. Dissecting the larynxes of hundreds of different animals he has traced the development from a simple valve to the most magnificent musical instrument in existence.

He has shown that not the anatomical structures but the conditions of life have determined the use of the larynx for voice. Animals living in open spaces (giraffes, antelopes) have no need for voices. Some higher animals have all the structures of the human larynx yet use no voice.

It was left to the creation of man to take all the parts of the respiratory tract, give them new functions and make them sing. But this was not yet the end. Greater brain power created the need for the highest form of communication from man to man, unknown to animals and lifting human beings to a level that exists nowhere else in nature.

Again, creation found new use for old structures. The mouth, the entrance for the digestive system, became the instrument for *speech*, the finest of all human achievements. This will be our story for the next chapter.

IV. *The Elements of Speech*

"In the beginning was the word."

We are not born with speech but, in a deeper sense, our real life as human beings begins with the moment when the first word leaves our lips. It takes us a year and often longer to reach this stage. The cry of our first days—a protest against a cold and hostile new world—becomes more variable and differentiated but for months it still takes the loving interpretation of the mother to identify the expressions of pleasure or anger, of hunger or pain.

Slowly we begin to experiment with sounds. We go through the "babbling" stage, producing an increasing variety of vocal combinations. We echo syllables in nonsensical repetition. We imitate speech sounds in clumsy distortion.

And finally the first word makes its appearance. Up to that point we have little to show that would make us superior to the higher animals. We are even more helpless and longer in need of the constant care of the mother.

We begin to prove our higher destiny when we try, for the first time, to stand up on our legs. But the moment that sets us really apart from all other beings is the birth of the first word.

From that hour on we belong to humanity. We need years to complete the miracle of fully developed speech. According to Dr. S. Ainsworth our vocabulary grows from 10-20 words at eighteen months to 50-250 words at the end of the second year and 800-900 words at the end of the third year. And it keeps growing through most of our life.

We learn to put words together, first in simple combinations, then in whole sentences. From the use of words as simple labels for persons and objects we graduate to their higher application: to express desires, to describe events, to define groups and categories, to formulate abstractions and ideas.

The growth of speech and language through childhood and adolescence is a fascinating subject, much too complex for the limitations of this book. We have to begin where adult speech has already become the powerful tool of communication.

Speech is voice or voiceless breath, modified by articulation. By *articulation* we understand the movements which change the shape and form of the cavities above the vocal cords. The throat, the soft palate, the tongue, the lips, singly or in groups, produce a tremendous variety of such changes which mold the air stream into the individualities of speech sounds.

Voice provides the level, the intensity and the range of speech. The average female voice in speaking is one octave higher than the male voice. Dr. Harvey Fletcher established the mean fundamental frequency of the male voice in vowels at 124 double vibrations per second (corresponding to the B of the musical scale) and for the female voice at 244 (the b). But these values vary with the types of voices, deep and high ones.

The average speech level of an individual can be determined by listening to his speech and comparing it with tuning forks or better whistles of standard pitch. It requires a good ear and much practice.

In actual speaking we constantly deviate in small intervals—thirds or fourths—from our basic level. In addition, the voice level of our speech is raised or lowered by emotional changes.

Fear, excitement, anger, joy and many other emotions push our voice up or down, far from the level we use in contentment and equanimity.

Out of the raw material of the voice we form, by modification of the air stream, the speech sounds that constitute the elements of the spoken word. We use a large number of them, many more than the letters of the alphabet we learned in school. To discuss the mechanics of each sound would lead us too deep into the underbrush of phonetics. If you want to acquire a more complete knowledge of this interesting field you should turn to one of the books you find in the bibliography.

We shall confine our discussion to the general principles that rule the production of speech elements. For this purpose we can use the well-known classification of vowels and consonants. But you have to keep in mind that we are going to describe speech sounds, not the letters of the printed or written alphabet.

Vowels, in the definition of Dr. Grant Fairbanks, are "voiced speech sounds in which the vocal cord tone is selectively modified as it passes through the resonance cavities of the throat and head."

The ability of changing voluntarily the shape of lips and mouth is a rather late achievement in evolution. Reptiles, birds have no lips and cheeks, only rigid structures of the mouth. Of the mammals, the apes have muscular mouth cavities of great pliability, but only man has learned to control them to the degree of changing the resonating qualities.

In describing vowels we are confronted with a difficulty we shall encounter frequently in this chapter: that the letters of the conventional alphabet are quite insufficient to identify vowels and consonants clearly. In languages with phonetic spelling, like Italian, the letters A E I O U conform, to a high degree, to the actual speech sounds. The English language is blessed with a grammar of great simplicity and with a vocabulary the richness of which satisfies the scientist and the poet alike, but it is cursed with an antiquated and completely erratic spelling.

The child, luckily, begins to speak long before he learns to read. He is not bothered by the fact that in saying "father," "stranger," and "salt" three different vowel sounds are used although the same letter of the alphabet appears in the printed word.

But the adult who has lost the ability of picking up language by ear and who needs books for the learning of a new tongue finds this discrepancy between symbol and sound very confusing.

As an added complication, the English language is rich in *diphthongs*, combinations of two different succeeding vowels. Here, too, the spelling gives no reliable clue.

To get some order into the great variety of vowel sounds one has tried to classify them according to articulatory movements in front, middle and back vowels. According to this classification typical front vowels are used in saying (and we quote again Dr. Fairbanks): "beat," "bit," "bait," "bat," "bet"; middle vowels in: "ask," "bird," "above"; back vowels in: "fore," "full," "fall," "hot," "calm."

Acoustically speaking, all these sounds are mixtures of a basic frequency, the fundamental, with a number of overtones or partials. In case you have forgotten, we discussed these terms in the last chapter.

Widening or narrowing of the mouth or throat changes the resonating properties of the cavities above the vocal cords. This makes it possible to create a great variety of fundamental-partial mixtures, resulting in different vowel sounds.

The overtones of vowels are mostly of the harmonic type. With modern equipment for sound analysis one has been able to register up to thirty-five different overtones in a single vowel sound.

Consonants are produced by a different mechanism. The

air stream is deflected, hindered or interrupted by obstacles we put into its way. We call the places where such obstacles are created the *zones of articulation.* There are three of them. The first zone lies between the lips, or between lower lips and upper front teeth. Consonants in this group are: P, B, W, Wh, F, V, M.

The second zone is found between front teeth, tip of the tongue and the hard palate behind the teeth. In this group are: T, D, Th, R, L, S, Sh, Zh, Y, N.

In the third zone are the sounds formed by the back of the tongue and the soft palate. To this group belong: K, G, Ng (as in "long").

Another classification of consonants can be gained by considering the type of obstruction they require. If a complete interruption of the air stream is needed we call these sounds *plosives*, because the air pressure is first built up behind the obstruction and then suddenly released in a tiny explosion. B and P are formed in this manner by the lips, T and D by the tip of the tongue and the hard palate, K and G by the back of the tongue and the soft palate.

If the air stream is not completely interrupted but forced through a narrow passage we call the resulting sounds *fricatives.* If you speak F, V, Th, S, Z, H you can feel and hear the air hissing through the narrow slits at the various points of formation.

Some consonants are spoken with a *gliding* movement, like W. They are half consonant, half vowel in character.

A third classification is based on the presence or absence of vocal cord vibration. We call these consonants *voiced* or *voiceless.* If you pronounce first a P and then a B you can feel the vibration of the cords, by placing your finger at the bottom of your mouth, in the B while they are absent in the P.

To the group of voiced consonants belong: B, D, G, V, Z; to the voiceless ones: P, T, K, F, S, Sh.

The *nasal sounds* are in a category by themselves. All speech sounds of the English language, with the exception of three are spoken with a raised soft palate. In this position the air stream is prevented from reaching the nose and is directed into the mouth. In three speech sounds the palate is lowered, thus opening the door into the nose: in M, N and Ng (as in string). In M the lips close the way through the mouth, in N tongue and hard palate, in Ng the back of the tongue and the soft palate. If you place your finger tip at the outside of the nostrils you will feel the vibration in these nasal sounds.

In French the vowels preceding nasal consonants are spoken with nasality too—one of the reasons why a good French pronunciation is so hard for English-speaking people.

So far, we have given you just the bare outline of the mechanics of speech sounds. Most likely, you are already quite bewildered by the complexity of a process that seems so simple when we use it in daily speech. Still, you can thank your lucky stars that you were born into one of the Western languages. There is no end to the variety of composite speech movements, from double stops in African languages, glottal stops in Dutch, to side-of-the-tongue sounds in Japanese.

In North Chinese groups of speech sounds may give four completely different meanings if spoken with changed intonation.

If we apply our acoustical knowledge to the consonants, we find that the partials or overtones which give them their characteristic color belong—in contrast to the vowels—more to the class of noises. The fricatives (like S or F) have particularly high frequencies in their overtones.

In analyzing speech frequencies one has found that the higher frequencies are very important for the intelligibility of speech. One can filter all frequencies under 500 out of speech and still obtain understandable communication, but the high frequencies cannot be eliminated without resulting in blurring. This explains the difficulties of the patient with a deafness that affects the acuity of the hearing nerve. In this type of deafness

—for instance, in old people—the high frequencies are the first ones to suffer. Although music can still be enjoyed to a certain degree, the understanding of speech deteriorates increasingly because of the loss of the high-frequency zone.

All the mechanisms we have so far discussed are part of the so-called normal voice and speech production. We say "so-called" because there is no man alive who fulfills in speech and voice all the requirements of normal function. Even the finest singers and speakers manage, at best, to come near to what we have to consider as perfect and, therefore, normal function.

In the field of speech sounds many outside influences modify the mechanics of vowels and consonants. Regional customs in the form of dialects and local speech habits lead to omission and modulation of speech sounds or to the substitution of "normal" sounds by others. The whole melody and inflection can be involved, creating new local "normalities" that would be irregular elsewhere. Think only of the Southern "drawl" or the New England "twang." In the case of the latter the characteristic voice of the Yankee is produced by a constriction of the glottis and by contraction of the lower part of the throat. You can produce the same effect by placing the flat hand against the region above the voice box and pressing hard upward and backward.

A famous example of the willful substitution of speech sounds is *ventriloquism.* This form of artificial speech has always intrigued scientists. In 1772 the French Abbé de la Chapelle wrote the first treatise on ventriloquism. His rather obscure explanations were vastly improved by Flatau and Gutzmann—two pioneers in our field—who in 1894 published the results of careful studies of ventriloquists.

Even now, with ventriloquism having become a fad through the popularity of such radio shows, many people have rather fantastic notions about the mysterious origin of the ventriloquist's voice. Actually, the ventriloquist uses the same vocal organs as we do. But his biggest problem is to avoid all speech sounds of the frontal zone of articulation since any movement of the lips would instantly destroy the illusion he tried to create. He has to learn to use contractions of the throat and soft palate together with retraction of the base of the tongue to produce substitute speech sounds. From these maneuvers the voice of the ventriloquist acquires the typical pressed quality, so familiar to the radio fan.

Now, let us for a moment return to a problem we touched already: the relationship between speech sounds and the written or printed word.

All Western languages use systems of letters to build up words. Some languages, like Italian, approach nearly the ideal of identifying the spoken sound by a letter of the alphabet. For the student of French or German it is already more difficult to guess from the combination of letters used the correct pronunciation. But English has one of the most irregular and unprecise ways of defining the spoken word by alphabetical symbols. The discrepancy between spelling and pronouncing is very great in our language.

You have only to look at the following pairs of words to realize how often similar spelling is used for different pronunciations, or the same sound spelled differently:

pr*i*de—b*i*rth	l*au*gh—bec*au*se	*g*eneral—a*g*ain
f*a*ther—d*a*nger	g*oo*d—m*oo*n	lo*ng*—da*ng*er
r*ea*ch—d*ea*th	*y*ou—tr*y*	*wh*ole—*wh*ite
s*ou*l—*ou*t	c*ow*—bl*ow*	*u*nder—t*u*tor

This system—or should one rather say confusion—of spelling is one of the main reasons why 10-14 per cent of the children in the U.S. have difficulties in learning how to read. To co-ordinate a group of letters to a spoken word is easier for a child in a language with phonetic spelling. It is very difficult in English and can be mastered only by the look-and-see method which stresses the grasping of the whole word as a unit.

For the purpose of speech analysis and research a *phonetic alphabet* that uses different symbols for each speech sound would be a great help. Many such phonetic alphabets have been constructed. The best so far, and most widely accepted one, is the alphabet on which the International Phonetic Association has agreed. It uses 63 symbols for consonants and 28 for vowel sounds. According to Dr. Grant Fairbanks, at least 41 of these symbols (15 for vowels and 26 for consonants) are necessary to identify the speech sounds of American English.

Most of the larger dictionaries employ their own simplified phonetic system to indicate the pronunciation of a word but in each the number of such "letters" is larger than the 26 of the alphabet. All phonetic alphabets have the same limitations: nobody has yet devised a system that includes all the speech sounds used in all human languages. Human speech is too rich to be fully mirrored in printed symbols. No letter can ever do justice to the countless varieties which the habits of language, country, region and individuality impress on spoken sounds.

Before closing this chapter a last word should be said about the *control of the speaking voice by the brain.* All actions and functions of our body can be grouped into voluntary and involuntary ones. For instance: we move arms or legs by voluntary muscular contractions, but our heart beats rhythmically, independent of our will.

The involuntary functions are under the supervision of the so-called autonomic nervous system, consisting of a number of centers in the brain and a chain of nerve control points in the body.

Voluntary actions are controlled by centers which are located on the surface of the two halves of the brain. The gray *cortex*, as the outer layer of the brain is called, contains the centers for body movements and sensations.

Breathing, the driving force of the vocal organs, is a mixed voluntary-involuntary function. If we sleep or, while awake, pay no attention to our breathing it goes quite automatically in a steady rhythm. The *respiratory center*, like the automatic steering of a modern plane, keeps the breathing going. But the pilot, the cortex, can at any time take over. We are able to breathe with voluntary control at any desirable depth provided that we respect the oxygen needs of the body. We cannot suppress breathing beyond a relatively short period.

In ordinary speaking, we are not aware of our breathing movements but the actor is, at least when he tries to arrange a long passage in artistically satisfying breathing periods. The student of speaking or singing may begin with exercises for voluntary breathing control. The singer when studying a part uses conscious breathing. With improved technique, with greater familiarity with an aria, breathing again becomes automatic. In short: breathing is an automatic process most of the time but we can assume conscious command whenever we wish.

The brain control of *speaking* is as complicated as speech itself. The experts who have devoted a lifetime to the research in brain functions are still in doubt about many details. For our practical purpose a few facts are sufficient that most of the scientists agree upon.

To be able to speak we need centers which receive outside messages. We hear the speech of others and relay the acoustical sensations to the brain by the pathways of hearing. The same happens to visual impressions if we look at objects or at reading material. All these incoming messages must be understood and interpreted. This takes place in a *sensory speech center* in the temple region of the brain, described first and named after a German psychiatrist Wernicke.

Then, with the help of other centers in the "thinking area" of the brain that store memories and promote associations, the message we intend to send out by the spoken word is prepared. Now, the actual act of speaking can begin. This requires the concerted effort of many muscles that move lips, tongue, palate, throat, vocal cords and the machinery of breathing.

This complex mechanism is under the control of a *motor speech center* in the frontal region of the brain surface. The French surgeon Paul Broca determined the localization of this center by a simple and ingenious method. In a number of cases which had shown loss of motor speech after a stroke he looked, after the death of the patient, for the area of brain damage. He drew outlines of the brain and of the field of destruction on sheets of tracing paper. By putting a pile of such tracings on top of each other he found that they all had in common a small area on the left side of the frontal brain and concluded that there the center of speech movements must be located.

To illustrate the whole process by a simple example: somebody asks you how much two times two is. Your ears receive the sound of the words and telegraph the question as acoustic impressions to the brain where it is delivered to Wernicke's sensory speech center. With the help of other centers of the "thinking area" the question is understood, interpreted, the correct answer "four" prepared (by reviving schoolday memories) and finally relayed to Broca's motor speech center. Under its command all your vocal organs begin at once to work as a team with the result that the loud answer is produced in the form of a spoken word.

The nerve fibers of the brain, on their way from the centers to the spinal cord and from there to the muscles, cross over to the other side. Thus, the left side of the brain serves the right side of the body and vice versa.

In most people, particularly in right-handed ones, speech is controlled from the left side of the brain. A damage to the motor region of this side of the brain—for instance, by the internal bleeding of a stroke—has very tragic consequences: in addition to the loss of motion in the right arm or leg the patient will lose speech if Broca's center is involved.

To repeat: this is a very sketchy outline of a complicated

and highly controversial subject. But it will help, together with everything we discussed in this chapter, to confirm the conviction we expressed in the beginning—what a miracle the first word, the first sentence we speak really is. How many organs have to work in finest co-ordination to make speech possible. No wonder that speech is the privilege of man, the highest form of organized life on earth.

Speech originated as an instrument for simple communication. Primeval man when he learned to speak must have been satisfied and proud to utter short sentences, expressing facts, reports, commands, desires and emotions.

Like the child's talk the speech of mankind has grown through the eons. It has become a tool for innumerable uses. This variety of a fully developed instrument, the possibilities and requirements of its professional use and the integration of voice and personality will be the subjects of the next chapter.

V. *Characteristics of the Speaking Voice*

One of the advantages the student of the human voice enjoys is that he hardly ever gets bored if he listens to somebody else. Of course, he shares the common preference for the interesting, the entertaining, the witty fare for his ears. But even if the play is dull, the sermon overlong, the political speech full of platitudes, the radio program below his level or the dinner conversation banal he does not suffer too much. Unwilling to follow what is said he concentrates on the "how." He analyzes voices.

To do so means to turn one of the greatest burdens of modern life into an enjoyable asset. For any man who prefers to think his own thoughts the flood of words that engulfs us everywhere, from loudspeakers, through windows and walls, is almost intolerable unless he develops some kind of escape mechanism. To analyze the "how" to escape from the "what" would have its own justification.

But it is much more than an intellectual self-defense. To listen to voices can teach us a great deal about the speaker, his background, his social and professional standing, his health, his personality.

To a certain degree we all analyze voices without being aware of it. We speak of pleasant, sincere, affected, monotone, irritating voices. But our judgment is based either on one outstanding voice symptom or on a general superficial impression.

The speech and voice therapist has to learn to examine a voice as the physician does the body: to consider each function separately, take note of all deviations from the normal and finally synthetize all findings into one overall diagnosis.

If we see a voice patient for the first time we let him talk and read, watching all the time the "how" more than the "what." To get some order into our impressions we try to ascertain a number of basic facts:

We have to determine his general background; country of origin, regional characteristics, social level, educational and professional standing;

We try to learn as much as possible about the basic features of his individual speech and voice;

We watch for all clues his voice may give us to his character and personality;

We use our knowledge of the voice requirements for the type of work of the patient to form an opinion on his aptitude for his job or occupation;

We note all abnormalities of speech and voice as the basis of our diagnosis of our patients' troubles.

We shall follow the same route in this chapter with the exception of the last point which belongs to a later part of the book when we come to the disturbances of the voice.

We hope to stimulate your interest in this kind of analytical hearing. No book can be a substitute for the trained ear. By concentrated listening to voices in conversation, on the radio, in movies and plays, one can develop a high degree of judgment of people through analysis of their voices if one knows where the clues are.

Much of our knowledge in this field has come from the study of the disturbed voice. As in all branches of medicine the abnormal is often a good starting point for the understanding of normal function.

We like to think of ourselves as individualities, unique and different from all others. Actually, we are, to a large extent, the products of our surroundings. The country we belong to, the place where we live, our social and professional background, our psychological type determine countless details of our personality.

Listening to the speech of a man teaches us a great deal about these formative factors. It is easy to notice whether a man speaks his mother tongue or an adopted language. We are familiar with the characteristics of dialects that betray the part of the country a man comes from. If he has changed his place of residence frequently the task becomes more difficult. Years ago, an interesting radio program, run by an expert in linguistics, enjoyed great popularity. By talking to guests for a few minutes he almost invariably was able to bring out their place of birth within a radius of a few hundred miles, to tell them where they went to college and to trace their subsequent residential itinerary.

The farther removed we are from the residence of another person, the more difficult it is for us to discover his personal speech and voice habits under the layers of group characteristics.

A tourist from Atlanta, Georgia, in Rome will appear to Italian ears as an English-speaking person; in London he will be an American whose speech differs from the "king's English"; in New York people will immediately recognize the Southern drawl; in his country house in Georgia his speech will stamp him as a city man for the ears of the rural "woolhead." Only in Atlanta will he be on his home ground with his voice. There the individualities of his speech will stick out even for less trained observers.

Social level, racial temperaments, professional surroundings and many other influences leave their mark on speech and voice. What may be the expected pattern in the speech of one group would be abnormal in another one. The speech and voice characteristics of a lonely fisherman would be as incongruous in the mouth of a big-city lawyer as hunting clothes on Park Avenue.

Having thus cleared away the group characteristics we can turn to the analysis of the basic components of individual speech. A very good way of training one's ear to perceive the finer details of speech is to listen to the radio. There a great variety of disembodied voices is offered at all times with no visual crutches to help us in making our observations. Voice therapists make frequent use of *recordings* of the voices of their patients. They can be played many times, permitting concentration on different features. The judgment of one therapist can be submitted to the critical review of others who never saw the patient. Recordings can be used to compare the voice or speech of the same individual at different times.

Analysis of a speaking voice includes appraisal of both articulation and voice. Outside of speech defects where, of course, examination of all elements of articulation stands in the foreground, the importance of articulation is somewhat overrated. In judging speaking voices, voice deserves much more attention than it usually gets. In schools, training centers for teachers and ministers, in drama departments the qualities of the voice are too often neglected in favor of articulation, a heritage from the times when "elocutionists" taught everywhere an artificial declamatory style of bygone days.

Articulation carries only the factual contents of the spoken message, while voice conveys the whole gamut of emotions and the impact of personality.

With the neglect of voice culture in our education and training it is no wonder that a clear, pleasant and impressive voice has become a rarity in adults and sticks out of the flood of deformed, distorted and ill-fitting voices that surround us everywhere. It is characteristic that one good book on voice lists only the negative qualities one should watch for in speaking voices: breathy, harsh, hoarse, nasal. We hear them constantly.

In examining voices one has to proceed, as the doctor does when he examines a patient: to follow a certain routine.

Every voice therapist has his own classification of basic voice elements. Dr. R. Curry suggests: pitch, intensity, duration and quality. The first three are specific, the last one too general for concise observations. Dr. P. Moses uses a more detailed qualification which permits a systematic approach to the analysis of speaking voices. His scheme has the added advantage that it is easy to remember because the main terms all begin with an R. His "5 R's" are: respiration, range, register, resonance and rhythm.

We have met *respiration* frequently as the driving force of the voice. Every speaker has a characteristic way of breathing life into his words. Whether we make conversation, address a crowd, recite Shakespearean periods, tell an amusing story, our breathing can be adequate, fitted to the occasion, effortless or pressed, exaggerated, insufficient.

Respiration mirrors the emotional equilibrium at all times, as you probably have found out when you had to make your first speech. At home, in the quietude of your study, the sentences of your manuscript sounded fine when you tried them out. But on the stage, under the pressure of tension or stage fright, you were suddenly confronted with the problem of "catching" your breath for effective delivery. The inspiration-expiration rhythm can be upset one way or the other, inadequate or too much pressure being used, disrupting the message of the sentence.

Range comprises the deviations from the basic pitch, that create the melody of our speech. We have discussed pitch in the last chapter. The range of our speaking voice constitutes normally the lower third of the whole compass we can employ in singing. In listening to individual voices we have to watch both the basic pitch and the range. A voice may be pitched too high or too low; it may exhibit an unusually wide range or be limited to a level of flat monotony.

The change of our moods influences particularly basic pitch and range. In excitement or sudden fear the pitch goes up and the range may widen, while depression lowers the pitch and narrows the range to a dull lifelessness.

We shall have more to say in the next chapter about the *registers* of the singing voice. Suffice it to say here that the adult speaking voice is a blend of the deep, the chest register and the high one, the head register. We shall discuss the change of voice in adolescence in the next chapter, and the abnormalities of this process, resulting in separation of the registers, and the constant use of a wrong register in Chapter XII.

Resonance as we have seen before is a basic function of voice production. Every change in the form and shape of the resonating cavities influences the quality and character of the voice sounds. The trained ear can detect many deviations from normal resonance and can even determine the exact place of tightness or weakness in the resonating cavities. An outstanding example of such change of resonance is nasality of speech, caused by momentary or permanent relaxation (or paralysis) of the soft palate. The reasons for this occurrence are manifold as we shall see.

Finally, *rhythm* of speech is a rather complex phenomenon. Rhythm rules our life in many ways and finds its expression in speech too. The language we speak provides the basic rhythm, from the fast delivery of the Latins to the slow pace and hesitant grouping of words by the Northern races. Our station in life puts its stamp on the speed, the duration of the individual sounds, the grouping and stressing of words in our speech. The speech rhythm—and the rhythm of life—of a peasant and of a salesman are different. The small-town man differs likewise from the big-city dweller, the minister from the lawyer, the slow-thinking from the quick-minded.

We shall meet all the basic features of speech again when we come to the discussion of voice and speech disturbances in the last part of the book. At this point, we just want to stress again the importance of getting away from generalized description of voices by terms which have no specific meaning and of learning to analyze each single factor that goes into the making of a voice.

Having satisfied ourselves about the "how" of a man's way of speaking we can then try to answer the "why." With voice being one of the most characteristic functions of an individual this question leads us logically to the connection between voice and personality.

Dr. P. Moses whom we mentioned before has studied the subject extensively. He believes that it is possible by what he calls "creative hearing" to find out a great deal about the personality and personality problems of a man. By watching closely every detail of the speaking voice a composite picture emerges of personality traits, moods, attitudes and many other facets of the personality.

As in all studies of human psychology great experience is required to pick the really important data out of a mass of detail and to assign the correct significance to each symptom.

One difficulty of identifying the meaning of each observable symptom lies in the fact that it is frequently what the psychologists call ambivalent: it can be interpreted in a positive or a negative way.

A man who speaks in a slow rhythm may be sure of himself, thinking carefully before he ventures an opinion, weighing his words before he lets them out. He may be slow of speech because he is slow of thinking, dull-witted, or shy and hesitant. Or he may affect this mode of speaking out of an exaggerated opinion of his own importance, speaking constantly in pronunciamentos to which everybody should pay close attention. In short: he may be a born leader, a stupid man or a pompous ass.

Fastness of speech, on the other hand, may be the expression of a mind overflowing with ideas or just the mirror of a shallow personality that releases a stream of superficial small talk without inhibition or criticism.

It is in the field of voice disturbances that knowledge of the voice-personality relationship can be a great help to better understanding of the causes of such conditions.

Take for instance a person with a rather deep-speaking voice. This will be his natural pitch if he belongs to the class of bassos. It may be the expression of great authority. The preacher, the judge, the doctor, the king on the stage, everybody who represents authority, tends to speak with the true pathos of deep sonorous voices. Such people will have no voice troubles since they use their voice at a genuine pitch, fitting the personality and the occasion.

But if we see a patient with voice trouble such as hoarseness after short periods of speaking and note that his voice is produced on an abnormally deep level we have to consider a number of possible causes: chronic laryngitis and other organic causes, lack of tension or weakness of the cords, glandular imbalances. But we will keep in mind the possibility that the patient has lowered his voice, consciously or subconsciously, to create the impression of an authority he actually does not possess. The young minister, teacher, district attorney are frequently the victims of this pseudo-pathos that wants to conceal the inner immaturity.

A loud voice may be the expression of energy and confidence as well as the product of a primitive mind without self-criticism.

The absence or exaggeration of nasality is another indicator of moods and emotions. A group of doctors at the New York Hospital (T. Holmes, H. Goodell, St. Wolf, H. Wolff) has recently published the results of an extremely interesting study of the influence of emotions on the mucous membranes of the nose and the deeper respiratory tract. By observing their patients constantly for weeks and months, sometimes from hour to hour, they could demonstrate that any change in the mood, any increase or decrease of tensions, fears or apprehensions is paralleled in the obstruction or widening of nasal passages, bronchi and bronchioles. They may shrink in sudden fear or produce in prolonged anxiety the pattern of "shutting off." It stands to reason that such changes influence voice resonance and vary the degree of nasality.

We could go on like this—and the temptation is great—for a long time without exhausting all possibilities. We would have to speak of melody of speech, exactness, accents and stresses and many other features of the speaking voice. The limited selection we presented should be sufficient to impress on you three facts:

That there exists an intimate connection between voice and personality, emotional balance, moods, passing and lasting emotions.

That a correct interpretation can be reached only with great care; by consideration not of one single outstanding symptom but only by a synthetic evaluation of all available details. This requires great experience and understanding. Psychological analysis of the personality by any approach is not the intellectual parlor game by which it is so frequently abused these days.

Finally, that—with these limitations in mind—listening to voices can teach each of us a great deal. It is a new and very promising field. Many questions are still to be answered, much research to be done on a large scale, many doubts to be cleared away. But in the end, we might be able to prove that vocal analysis is a new and valuable tool for the struggle with the age-old endeavor: to understand the human mind.

And now, let us turn to a subject of immediate practical application: the specific requirements for the different uses of speech and voice.

Much too little attention has been paid to this problem. Every year, thousands of young people embark on careers that are founded on the use of the voice without giving a thought—or being advised to get an opinion—to their aptitude for such work. It cannot be emphasized too much that everybody at this crossroad of life should get a complete check-up by a competent examiner. The vocal organs should be investigated for all kinds of possible organic abnormalities, such as obstructions of the nose, sinus troubles, adenoids, tonsillitis, allergies, asthma. The larynx should be inspected and shape, appearance, motility and closure of the vocal cords determined. Finally, and most important of all, speech and voice should be tested by an expert who has been trained in this field and knows something about the working conditions of the voice in jobs and professions.

In this respect, very little work has been done. Aptitude tests almost invariably omit consideration of the voice.

Take the case of *salesmen*, for instance. The big department stores test their permanent employees carefully, train them in preparatory courses but pay no attention to the correct and efficient use of the voice. If you go through the busy sections of a large store you can hear all kinds of bad voices. The salesgirl who talks almost incessantly in noisy surroundings for eight hours a day, five days a week, easily develops voice troubles on the base of the constant abuse, pressure and strain. If you start your career in this field already with poor speech and voice habits you are a likely candidate for permanent disturbances.

The higher the qualities of goods to be sold, the greater the need for the persuasiveness of a pleasant voice. There you need more than great stamina of a voice that can produce quantities of speech without getting tired or hurt. It is the quality of a good sales voice—a voice which expresses your interest in your work—that counts.

What makes us so often buy things we did not intend to? Is it, as most employers believe—aside from the desirability of the object—the sales talk, the "what," or is it the influence of the voice, the "how"? One thing is certain: the overworked, overstrained voices we hear so often in stores and offices make us uncomfortable, create the wish to get out of earshot as fast as possible.

Switchboard operators with their long hours of constant talk work under the handicap of quantity too. In this type of work clearness of articulation counts, of course, foremost but good voice is essential for success. The big telephone companies know that very well. They are almost the only employers who put candidates for jobs through systematic training of speech and voice. In addition, they have created large laboratories where extensive research is being done on acoustic and phonetic problems.

Next to sales personnel and telephone operators, *teachers* of all kinds carry the heaviest load of speaking. Teaching puts a great strain on the voice, by the sheer quantity of speech alone. Teachers have to represent authority in front of a class that is often resistant, noisy and even belligerent. If they are born educators, with natural authority and a sound voice, their job is not too difficult. But only a minority can fulfill all these requirements. The result is frequently the use of a voice that is out of focus in pitch, function and economy.

Voice troubles are a typical occupational hazard of the teacher. Still, aside from watching faults of articulation, very little is done in the training of teachers to study and improve their voices. This is the more regrettable because teachers set standards by their own example. Their pupils pick up faulty speech and voice habits from the teacher while their own voices are still in the formative stage. In addition, the resistance we all feel if exposed to unpleasant and irritating voices endangers the relationship between teacher and pupil.

To watch and correct faults of articulation of teachers in training is not enough. Nobody should be permitted to choose the teaching profession without an examination and, if necessary, correction of his voice.

The higher the standards of professional speech are—both

in content and delivery—in any type of work, the less important the tolerance for great quantities of speech becomes and the more decisive the quality. But in these professions—such as the minister's, the lawyer's, the actor's, the lecturer's—psychological factors create special voice hazards. The tension, the responsibilities, the risks, the personnel problems combine to throw the speaker off his emotional balance. The importance of his voice for his career and success exposes him anyhow to the dangers of vocal hypochondria; and the neurotic conflicts, so frequent in these professions, have a preference for fixation on the voice.

As with the teachers, guidance in the use of the voice should form a main subject in the training of *ministers*. What they actually get is very little or nothing. Any voice therapist who had a chance to work with divinity students knows that their first sermons are very often quite an ordeal. Some ministers—even widely known stars of the pulpit—fight with their voices through their whole life. Nobody had ever analyzed their vocal equipment when they began to study. They have to speak in churches and temples with obstinate acoustics. The burden of representing moral authority in the upheavals and contradictions of modern society is rather heavy.

The "clergyman's throat"—as the voice troubles of the ministers have been called for generations—is not so often the result of a cold or laryngitis as the expression of poor training, faulty use and constant strain on the vocal organs. Expert guiding and advice during the years of training would go far to eradicate this scourge of the clerical profession.

While the minister uses voice to guide people, the task of *actors* is to imitate and recreate life in all its forms. This requires a tremendous flexibility and adaptability of the voice which only a few achieve. In addition, they have to master the technique of "projection," the ability to bridge the distance—sometimes very great—between the stage and the audience without changing or distorting the type of speech the play requires. Actors with a perfect speaking voice will be equally natural, audible and pleasant to your ears, whether you sit in the first row of the orchestra or high up in the balcony. Clarity of diction helps a great deal but the good use of the voice, equally well adapted to the character of the part as to the acoustic dimensions of the theater, decides the success.

In their difficult task, actors in the theater get effective help by visual assistance. Gestures, make-up, costume, scenery, contribute to creating the illusion of the play. *Radio actors* work without any of these props. By their voice alone they have to create the character they portray. If they play a king, a gangster, a businessman, the listener must get the full impact of the personality through the ear. This leads easily to an abuse of the voice which has ruined the career of many good actors. Although they have not to overcome the problem of voice projection—with the microphone permitting speech on conversational level—they suffer often from the conventions which radio-speaking has developed. Radio has created an overemotional type of its own that has spoiled our ears for the finer shadings of the speaking voice. The commentators, who speak with the voice of doom or hysteria, the announcers who must advertise the goods in exaggerated outbursts, to please the sponsor, the actors in soap operas who have to wade through the artificial emotions of daily catastrophes, they all have created a new audience which takes the extreme for the normal.

In our age of mass communications nobody can escape the influence of radio and television. The overexcited, overstrained voices that reach us constantly through countless loudspeakers set new patterns and fashions of speech and voice, particularly with the younger generation.

Everybody who works in radio has to convey his message through the medium of microphone and loudspeaker. One could write a whole book about the *microphone*, its impact on modern society, its possibilities and limitations and its effect on human voices.

The microphone has narrower limits in range and intensity than the human voice. If you speak through a microphone—as actor, politician, lecturer, preacher—you should be thoroughly familiar with the technique it requires. The microphone speaker must be able to express the whole variety of desirable emotions while respecting the limits of loudness where distortion or lack of response begin. Most radio speaking is done with directional microphones which are sensitive to any change of the position of the speaker. A turn of the head, a step to the side changes the effect of the voice for the listener.

The microphone has radically changed the impact of the human voice on our political life. It has become both a blessing and a curse. It has made possible the "fireside chat" where a voice can talk to millions in conversational tones. And it has served as a tool in the creation of mass hysteria by the voice of one man alone. Modern dictatorships have rediscovered the truth of a remark Gibbon made 175 years ago that "the mechanical operation of sounds, by quickening of the blood and spirits, will act on the human machine more forcibly than the eloquence of reason and honor."

Those of us who put the microphone to more peaceful pursuits overlook easily the effect of this mechanization of sound on the quality of the human voice. If we speak through a microphone the listener does not hear our voice, but a filtrate of our voice sounds through the medium of a complicated machinery. Apart from distortion which poor equipment produces we are at the mercy of the sound engineer. This modern Pygmalion can create voices, almost out of nothing, by the witchcraft of his panel.

He can blow up conversational speech to the dimensions of the arena. He can emphasize the lower or higher frequencies of our voice and thereby change its character completely. We have seen how important the overtones which range through the whole compass of audible sounds are to the quality and expressivity of the voice sounds we produce.

Finally, the microphone has become a crutch that threatens to destroy the art of free speaking. Most speakers have become so dependent on the assistance of the microphone that they are afraid to address a hundred listeners without it. Movie and television actors have lost the ability to project their voices and go through agonies when they want to appear in a play.

It is time that we learn again to use the natural force and power of our voices as our fathers did who thought nothing of speaking for an hour to an audience of a thousand and more without microphones. If we can do that only by reducing the daily flow of speech which engulfs us now to rarer and more important occasions we can only benefit from such rationing of words.

Of course, power and force can be overdone. The auctioneer, the barker at the country fair have to put a prolonged strain on their voices. Only few vocal cords can sustain it with impunity.

In this category the *voice of command* ranks high as particularly dangerous. The soldier who leads men has to use loud voice in short powerful bursts. His commands have to be sharp in articulation and clearly audible on the drill ground as well as in the field. They must carry the ring of absolute authority which men follow without questioning even under danger of life. The easiest but rather dangerous way of producing the penetrating command voice is to use the so-called *glottal stroke*, the forceful compression of the vocal cords which permits the explosive release of pent-up air. This leads to thickening of the cords or the formation of nodes which, in turn, necessitate even greater force for loud commands. The "fog-horn" voices of the top sergeant, of the oldtime sailing ship captain are sad examples of the ruining of voices by long abuse.

Training schools for officers and noncommissioned officers should include instruction in the proper use of the voice in their curriculum. Instead of insisting on harsh barking, the proper technique of starting with a soft attack and of stepping up sound in fast increase of volume—the way a good driver operates the gas pedal—should be taught.

There are many more different types of professional work requiring voice and speech, each with its own characteristic tasks and voice problems.

Altogether, it should be clear—even from this short survey—that no simple prescription can be given for a good speaking voice. The most important requirement for everybody who uses speech in his work is to retain and develop his personal normal voice. Very few of us manage to escape the distorting influences of modern life. Voices of normal pitch, melody, flexibility are as rare as normal feet in our shoe-ridden civilization.

The only way out of this deplorable situation is *preventive voice care* on the largest scale. Systematic training of teachers, examination and care of adolescent voices and advice before and during job and professional training would go a long way to prevent the damage to voices we experience now everywhere.

So far, we have bypassed the finest use to which the human voice can be applied: artistic singing. It deserves a chapter of its own.

VI. *Singing Voices*

A few can touch the magic string,
  And noisy Fame is proud to win them:—
Alas for those that never sing,
  But die with all their music in them!

Of the many thoughtful lines that Oliver Wendell Holmes, doctor and writer of "Autocrat" fame, has penned about the human voice, none have defined so simply the variability of the use of the singing voice: from the release of the inner music in song by most of us to the glories of artistic singing by a chosen few.

We begin to sing almost as soon as we learn to speak. In an artless childish treble we imitate the songs of our mothers. They have to be simple to fit our narrow range. The best we can do at our second year is to produce a compass of six half-tones. Slowly the range widens.

According to Dr. E. Froeschels who measured the range of hundreds of school children the normal range at six years reaches from b to a^1, at eight from a to c^2, at ten from g to d^2, at twelve from e to d^2 (almost two octaves).

The big chance comes with puberty. Up to then, the voices of boys and girls follow the same line. *Mutation*, as the *change of voice* is called, is the crossroads where male and female voices separate.

During puberty, the fast maturing sex glands release hormones into the bloodstream and stimulate the development of the secondary sex characteristics that distinguish the adult body from the child's. The change of voice is but one of the manifestations of this stormy period. In temperate zones it takes place in girls between twelve and fourteen years and in boys between thirteen and fifteen. In warmer climates it begins one to two years earlier, in the cold zones up to two years later.

The slow growth of the larynx in childhood is suddenly accelerated in puberty. The cartilages extend mostly in the anterior-posterior position. The Adam's apple assumes its prominence, the neck lengthens, and the larynx moves to the middle of the neck. The vocal cords grow by about ⅖ of an inch in the male and by ⅛ of an inch in the female. At the end of mutation the lower limit of the male voice has descended by an average of an octave while the upper limit has dropped by about a sixth. In girls both limits descend only one to two tones.

In the majority of boys the whole process develops very gradually with no appreciable break of the voice. Only a small percentage goes through the period of cracking or breaking, the "Henry Aldrich" voice. In these cases the change might come almost overnight and throw the co-ordination of the vocal muscles completely out of gear.

David Sarnoff—now president of the Radio Corporation of America—used to sing in a synagogue choir as a boy of fifteen, with a fine soprano voice. On the day before the high holidays —as told in an article in *Time* magazine—when he expected to earn one hundred dollars for his singing, his voice suddenly broke and deprived him of a much needed income. It started him on a famous business career.

No certain prognosis can be made from a boy's voice about the quality and type of voice that will develop. According to Dr. D. Weiss who wrote a comprehensive study of mutation, a child's soprano often becomes a baritone or basso while altos frequently develop into tenors. Caruso sang the alto in a church choir. Chaliapin was a soprano before mutation.

While the speaking voice settles in an average of three to six months—with one year being the extreme limit for normal development—the singing voice needs much more time for full development. This is of practical importance for the answer to a question we have to discuss very often with our patients: at what age serious vocal studies can be safely begun.

In this connection, a discussion has raged for hundreds of years whether or not singing should be permitted at all during the change of voice. Manuel Garcia fought for complete voice rest against Dr. Morel Mackenzie who believed that easy exercises would be helpful in the transition of the voice. But all experts agree that choir singing—the prevalent form of singing at that age—with its lack of individual control is very harmful. Schubert and Haydn lost their voices that way. Serious vocal studies should not be begun in boys before the age of eighteen to nineteen, in girls before seventeen.

The adult voice has a range of at least two octaves, but many trained voices extend over three octaves and more. We have to distinguish between physiological and musical range. While the first one includes all notes that can be produced by a person, the latter one is limited to the range of artistically satisfactory sounds.

By old tradition, male voices are classified as bassos, baritones, tenors; female voices as contraltos (and altos), mezzo-sopranos and sopranos. In Fig. 8 you find the average ranges of these six categories as determined by Dr. M. Nadoleczny through examination of six hundred singers.

The basic speaking pitch—marked by small horizontal lines—corresponds closely to the range of the singing voice. As we shall see later any marked discrepancy between voice type and speaking pitch is of great significance in voice disturbances.

The absolute range is greater in deep voices. Bassos have

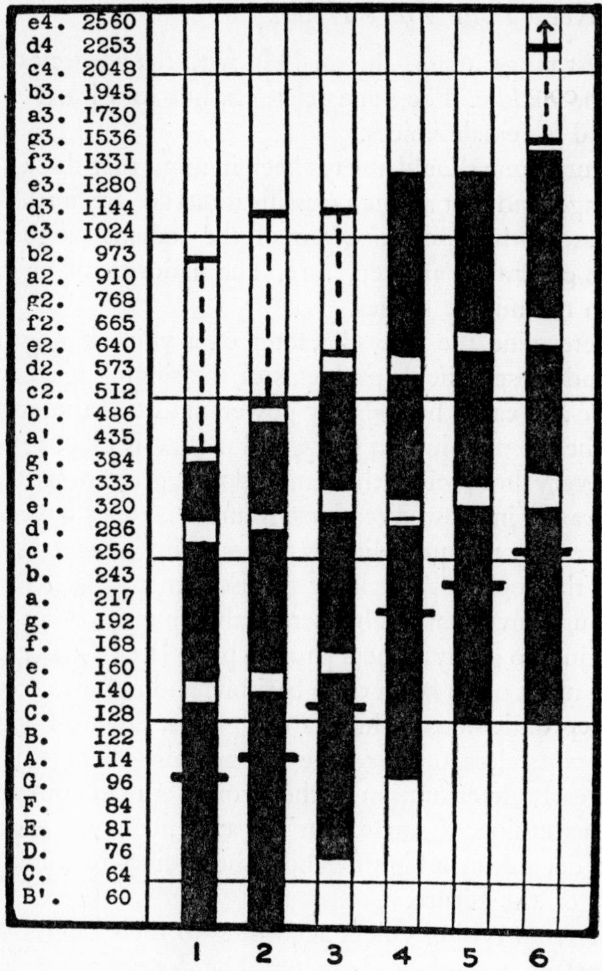

(Nadoleczny)

FIG. 8. The Ranges of the Human Voice
1. Basso. 2. Baritone. 3. Tenor. 4. Contralto.
5. Mezzo-soprano. 6. Soprano.

The gaps in the black columns indicate the approximate positions of the transitions between the registers. The dotted areas above the male voices are the falsetto voices. The dotted area above the soprano marks the whistle register.

The horizontal black lines indicate the average pitch of the speaking voice.

the widest range, tenors the smallest, with the baritones standing in the middle. The same relations, but to a lesser degree, are found in female voices.

Of course, one should always keep in mind that these figures are average, and that all such classifications are artificial. Really deep bassos—the *basso absoluto* of the Italians—high tenors and true contraltos are very rare. The majority of voices are found in the middle ranges.

To determine the true character of a voice is one of the oldest and most difficult problems of the singing teacher. It is not made any easier by the very powerful lure of the extremes. Since a heavy premium in glory and money is placed on very high or very low voices the temptation is great to extend the natural range in these directions. Many baritones have ruined their voices by masquerading as tenors, many a mezzo-soprano invaded the sopranos' territory to discover, too late, that one cannot jump over natural barriers with impunity. Some singers manage just to go by, others pay the price later. Chaliapin was actually not a basso but a deep baritone and ran into considerable voice difficulties in his maturer years. Some of the most famous contraltos of our time are actually mezzo-sopranos, and the early deterioration of their voices is a sad commentary on overextension of range. But the audiences roar if a singer hits the deep A or a high f^3, and nobody likes to think of the dangers of the future.

Aside from typing voices according to their ranges we can classify them as to their character. The *dramatic* and the *lyric* voices represent different types, both in voice and personality of the singer. Siegfried and Don Octavio, Eleonore and the Countess Almaviva pose not only very different vocal problems but ask for completely different personalities as well. The *buffi* have to be good comic actors and need flexible voices that permit a maximum of characterization. The true coloraturas are in a class by themselves. We shall discuss them when we come to the significance of registers.

Just in passing we should mention another type of voice that belongs to history: the *castrati.* The seventeenth and eighteenth centuries were the time of their greatest triumphs. Someone has figured that during that era in Italy every year four thousand boys were castrated to produce singers for the growing demands of church choirs and opera houses. Singing with the larynx of a child and the chest power of an adult, trained to a technical brilliance that will never again be duplicated, they were the great stars of their time. They made the Sistine Choir in Rome world famous; singers like Caffarelli, Farinelli, Senesino, Bernacchi commanded fees that would make our tenors blanch with envy. The *Orpheus* (Monteverdi and Gluck) and *Idomeneo* (Mozart) were written for castrates. Handel in London offered fabulous salaries to famous *castrati* for parts in his operas. With their passing from the musical scene the age of greatest singing came to a close to be followed by a new conception that valued dramatic truth in opera higher than smoothness of technique.

To succeed in opera is today the ambition of most singers. Too often the satisfaction of *concert work* is overlooked. In many European countries the artist who excels in the art of the lied, the oratorio is valued as highly as the operatic star (although the income is usually smaller). Music in America is relatively young. With the tremendous expansion of concert life that the last twenty years have brought, we begin to rely less on big opera stars and more on artists who master the different style of the concert hall. This is a very healthy symptom of our musical growth that will give new opportunities to many young artists.

A very strange by-product of modern mass communications is the *microphone voices* that become famous overnight and fade away after short bursts of a very profitable popularity. A few of them, like Sinatra's, exhibit at least a high degree of technical ability, but the majority of these so-called "voices" which sell millions of records are artificial creations of the amplifier that would sound tinny and shaky if the stars ever tried to sing without clutching a microphone.

Thousands of singers who do not make the grade in opera and concert, work as *soloists* in *church choirs*. This can be a very satisfactory occupation, both artistically and—on a modest level—economically. It is steady work, a rarity in the arts. It requires a great amount of musicality and versatility, and an easy facility in sight-reading.

Can the *type of a voice* be *determined by physical examination*? Teachers and singers have asked this question very often and, as usual, the experts disagree. Certain rules have been established but exceptions can be quoted to each of them. The singer is the instrument and the instrumentalist at the same time, and it stands to reason that his body structure should reflect the character of the voice as do the instruments, for instance, the violin and the cello.

To begin with the vocal cords, definite characteristics exist. Most singers with low voices have long and relatively thin cords, while the high voices have short and broad cords. The coloraturas have sometimes an incredibly small larynx with very short vocal cords.

The whitest cords are found in tenors and high sopranos while those of deep voices usually have a more pinkish tinge.

Dr. D. Weiss who examined a large number of successful singers believes that a definite body type can be associated with the high and low voices. According to him, singers with high voices have: round faces with short noses, a convex profile with small delicate details, short necks, round or quadratic chests, high palates with delicate soft palates; while the deep voices are characterized by: long faces with long noses, straight-line profiles with massive details, long and narrow necks, long and flat chests, broad palates with massive soft palates. A flat palate or a sharp angle between the floor of the mouth and the neck was rarely found in a singer with a good voice.

As long as we have not established these characteristics as certain it would be dangerous to design voices by physical characteristics alone. Still, it is astonishing how many singers fit into Dr. Weiss's scheme if one analyzes their body structure.

Fundamentally, singing is the same regardless of the purpose or grade. Whether we "sing" with our vocal cords in the speaking voice, or produce our best "bathroom tenor," our vocal organs follow the same basic laws of acoustics as the larynx of a Caruso. There is no need to repeat here the explanations of laryngeal function we gave in Chapter III. We want to limit our discussion to a few facts that pertain to *artistic singing.*

With *respiration* being the driving power of the larynx, good breathing is the basis of perfect singing. Artistic singing requires the ability to sing long musical phrases with all the accents and changes in intensity and pitch that the composer provided. No simple formula can be given that would fit all voices.

Graphic records of the chest and abdominal breathing of famous singers of the same voice category show great differences in the breathing mechanism. It is the task of the teacher to find out for each individual student by what teamwork of chest and abdomen the goal of every good singing can best be reached: to sing with the greatest economy of air. The less air used for a certain sound—whether piano or forte—the better the result will be.

This minimum consumption of air is possible only if all air is transformed into sound waves. Any attempt to obtain uncertain notes by enforced breathing—one of the most common faults of technique—will only lead to *waste of air*, the audible escape of unutilized air through the cords that is equally detrimental to the esthetic result as to the health of the voice. As Mackenzie already remarked, a good singer can sing a note without producing a flicker in the flame of a candle in front of the mouth.

In his classical study of the breathing mechanism of singers Dr. M. Nadoleczny found the smooth teamwork of chest and abdominal breathing characteristic of all good voices. Marked reliance on one type of breathing is almost always the sign of a poor technique that leads sooner or later to voice disturbances. The enforced chest breathing with lifting of the shoulders at the height of inspiration is particularly dangerous. It is a signal for the need of speedy correction before irreparable damage is done to the voice.

A great confusion surrounds the term *breathing support.* The *support* or, as the Italians call it, the *appoggio* is a special technique of slowing down the rate of expiration. Unfortunately, as it so often happens in discussions of singing, body sensations have been confused with the mechanism of function. Teachers have spoken of inspirational tension, or have claimed the forehead or the nose as the seat of the support for the voice.

We still cannot completely explain support in scientific terms. This much is certain: in true support the expiration is artificially slowed down by clinging as long as possible, after expiration has begun, to the position at the end of inspiration. Either the chest or the abdominal wall is kept at an extended position while the counterpart begins to contract. The abdominal support—leaving the abdominal wall and the flanks extended during the first phase of expiration—is generally considered the preferred method, and has been observed in top-ranking Italian singers. The "inspiratorial tension" that has been described by teachers and singers is a body sensation which should not be confused with the demonstrable slowing down of expiration that actually takes place. Expiration—whether slow or fast—is necessary for any kind of singing.

The use of subjective body sensations has a legitimate place in teaching. The student is often helped more by explanations in terms of such sensations than by physiological discourse. But the teacher who has to know the functional facts should always keep in mind that a valid analysis of mechanics of singing can be given only in terms of graphs, curves or by other means of scientific registration and observation.

Next to support no other detail of singing technique has suffered so much from misinterpretation as the term *register*. For generations, singers, teachers, doctors have formulated so many different explanations and classifications of registers that it is difficult to find a way through the maze of theories. Modern experimental research has brought some clarification.

Manuel Garcia who did not have our laboratory equipment has still presented one of the best definitions. In his *Traité Complet de L'Art du Chant* he wrote in 1841 he said: "By the word register we mean a series of succeeding sounds of equal quality on a scale from low to high, produced by the application of the same mechanical principle, the nature of which differs basically from another series of succeeding sounds of equal quality produced by another mechanical principle.

"Consequently, all the sounds which belong to the same register are of the same nature, regardless of changes in pitch or force to which they are submitted."

If a person with an untrained voice sings a downward scale from a high note, two breaks will be heard, that mark the limits of three different registers: the head, the middle and the chest register. The same occurs, of course, on an upward scale. On a descending scale the breaks occur at deeper points than on an ascending one. Each group of sounds has for the experienced ear a different quality.

It is the purpose of any training of the voice to make these transitional breaks disappear and to blend the whole range into one smooth unit. In a good voice it requires great practice to hear the transitions from one register to another. In the chart of Fig. 8 you find the average points of transition marked by small white spaces in the black columns.

High-speed cinematography has thrown some light on the registers. In the chest register the whole mass of the cords vibrates rhythmically, while in the head register only the inner margins of the highly tensed cords participate in the vibrations. At the same time the posterior parts of the cords remain firmly closed—the damping effect that prevents vibration so that only the anterior halves or thirds are left free to vibrate in the inner margins.

The ideal singing is done in a mixture of register characteristics in a *voix mixte*. Each tone of the compass receives a little of the color of the opposing registers in a mixture that varies from equal parts in the middle of the range to heavier coloring at the extreme ends.

The only case where a pure register is used in perfect singing is the coloratura who sings in a clear head register.

The chest voice uses more air than the head voice. The complete vibration of the whole mass of the cords requires a higher pressure of air to produce sounds of equal intensity as in the head register. In the chest voice the backward resonance can be felt at the breastbone. The vibrations in the chest have given the name to this register.

The male voices have on top of the head register the *falsetto* which even to the untrained ear has a distinctive quality of its own. The Italian masters of the early Bel Canto thought of it as an unnatural and therefore false voice—thence the name.

The falsetto is sung with only the foremost parts of the cords left free to vibrate at the margins, the rest being damped (see Plate II, C). It has less brilliance than the sounds of the head register. It can be used occasionally, but its continuous employment gives the voice an effeminate character.

The female voices have no real counterpart to the male falsetto, but the sopranos have a so-called *whistle register* on top of the head register (see Fig. 8). It has a shrill quality when used forte and sounds like a flute when piano. In artistic singing it is used only in high, fast staccato notes such as the f^3 of the "Queen-of-the Night" aria in the *Magic Flute*. (By some coincidence, Mozart's father Leopold was the first one to describe this register.) Like the falsetto, the whistle register is produced by marginal vibration in the anterior third of the cords which leave a tiny elliptic chink open.

In 1836, a French tenor, Gilbert Duprez, appeared in Paris with a new singing method he learned in Italy. In 1840, two doctors, Diday and Pérequin described this technique, calling it *voix sombrée*, *voix fermée* or *voix couverte*. The last name stuck and became the *covered voice* in English.

The controversy about the nature, the artistic value and the advisability of covered singing has been raging ever since. Many details are still obscure. Hundreds of papers have been written about it, but only lately—thanks to modern methods of sound analysis—have we begun to understand a little better the nature of covering.

The experienced ear can detect the degree of covering by the peculiar color it gives to the voice. It sounds somewhat darker and, at the same time, more penetrating. It is, therefore, particularly suited to singing with great dramatic expression. Wagnerian singers usually employ extensive covering of the voice. Under the influence of Wagner, Richard Strauss and the modern composers, covering has become, to a certain extent, the trademark of the German singer. The French do not like it much, and the Italians hate it. They prefer the *voce bianca*, the open voice. Play records of some great Wagnerian singer and of a first-class Italian in succession, and you will hear the difference in the vocal approach.

Covering has to be used with great care because, in its extreme form, it is hard on voices. Measurements of air volume have shown that the same note sung by the same singer uses in covered voice up to double the amount of air it uses in open singing. The reason for this result lies in the greater tension of the outer laryngeal muscles as well as of the inner ones both of which tense the cords.

The larynx is pulled downward in covering while in open singing it rises and falls with the pitch (although exceptions from this rule have been observed). Generally speaking, excessive *movements* of the larynx are typical for untrained or poor voices. In a mature singer they are a danger symptom, at least if the larynx moves in extreme, abrupt movements with the rise and fall of the pitch. The better trained the voice, the smaller the changes in position of the larnyx in singing from low to high or vice versa.

In the last chapter we mentioned the *coup de glotte* or *glottal stroke*. The term is used to describe the hard attack of a note by a sudden forceful compression of the cords with an explosive release of air. It is one of the most pernicious habits a singer can acquire, leading to formation of nodes, thickening of the cords and hemorrhages into the cords.

The singer has to learn to attack even the most powerful fortissimo with a soft beginning. In high-speed cinematography the difference can be clearly seen. In soft attack the cords begin already to vibrate before they come in contact with each other. In the glottal stroke the cords are squeezed together with a frightening force until they are suddenly blown apart by the mounting air pressure. Even strong vocal cords cannot stand this treatment for any length of time without suffering serious and often irreparable damage.

There is one exception to the general condemnation of the glottal stroke. In *staccato* singing a form of glottal stroke is used to produce the sharp interruptions of sound that characterize it. But in good staccato the glottal stroke which starts each note is well controlled and done with a minimum of pressure to avoid damage to the cords.

A well-trained voice exhibits always a certain amount of *vibrato* that gives the sounds more life and expression. By vibrato, we understand small rhythmical changes, both in pitch and volume. These oscillations of no more than half a tone and two to three decibels are more noticeable in forte tones than in piano. They take place at the rate of about six to seven per second.

If the wavering becomes excessive—up to twelve times per second—it is called *tremolo*, a greatly feared symptom of poor or deteriorating voices. It happens frequently in "throaty" voices and may be due to overtenseness of the muscles which creates a vibrating trembling in the throat, the tongue and sometimes even the jaw.

One factor that influences singing voices gravely is not so well known: the *standard pitch* used in tuning the instruments of the orchestra. If we read a score by Bach or Mozart we usually assume that the notes they wrote are the same we hear today when their works are performed. Actually, pitch has constantly risen in the last three hundred years. The old organ builders in the seventeenth century were the first to raise the standard pitch (Diapason) of the a^1 in order to save material by shorter pipes. From their pitch of 375-400 the a^1 rose at the time of Mozart and Handel to 420. In the nineteenth century the pitch became still higher until in 1859 a French commission fixed the "diapason normal" at 435 double vibrations per second. While all Europe accepted this as a standard pitch, the English continued to force the pitch until it had reached the peak of 458. The famous German violinist Joseph Joachim complained to Mackenzie that he had to start tuning up his violin eight weeks before a concert in London to prevent injury to the instrument by a sudden change.

Finally, an international agreement fixed the standard pitch at 435. This figure is still used in most textbooks although in the meantime a new change has taken place.

Unfortunately, in the last twenty-five years orchestras, especially in America have again begun to raise the pitch because it gives the woodwinds and, to a lesser degree, the other instruments a greater degree of brilliance. We hold now at 440 which was accepted in 1939 by an international conference in London. The U.S. Bureau of Standards in Washington, D.C., broadcasts daily a radio signal of 440 double vibrations per second as a standard a^1.

The sufferers of this development are the singers. Instruments can be tuned or built to conform to a higher pitch, but the human vocal cords remain the same. Mozart, Beethoven are played and have to be sung almost half a tone higher than the composers heard it. The b^2 flat that Leonore has to throw with full force at the threatening Pizarro, the c^3 that rings through the end of Constance's big aria and many similar hurdles of the operatic race course are now even more neck-breaking than they used to be for the singers of a more considerate time.

With the exception of the contraltos, all singers would be in favor of returning to the classical pitch. Audiences would be benefited too since they would be exposed to less of the shrieking we hear now so often.

There is hardly a chance to reverse a trend that has become universally accepted. But, at least, singers should unite in putting a stop to any further attempts to raise the standard pitch. No brilliance of the orchestra can compensate for the ruin of voices that follows each new upward change of pitch.

With the conclusion of this chapter we have come to the end of the first part of this book in which we discussed the normal speaking and singing voice.

The next five chapters will deal with medical matters: hygiene of the vocal organs, treatment of diseases that affect the voice directly or as a complication.

VII. *Keep Your Voice Healthy*

THE GREEKS HAD A WORD FOR IT, AND WE STILL USE IT TODAY. *Hygiene*, the science which deals with the preservation of health, has become a powerful force in the age-old struggle of mankind for a longer and happier life.

In the public domain, the rules of hygiene, as enforced by ordinances and regulations, health departments and the medical profession, govern countless aspects of our daily lives and—with the exceptions of a few crackpots—we willingly co-operate. Yet when it comes to personal hygiene, quite a different situation prevails. Years of study of patients and people in general have convinced us that personal hygiene consists, to a large extent, of advice freely given and rarely followed. And, as a rule, those who dispense the advice are not much better in living according to their own teaching.

To no group should the preservation of physical health be more important than to the men and women who make professional use of their speaking and singing voice. They are more vulnerable to any impairment of the vocal organs in particular, and—due to the nature of their work which brings them into constant contact with large numbers of people—they are more susceptible to infections in general than the rest of us. Furthermore, the risk of temporary or permanently debilitating effects of sickness becomes greater as specialization in the use of the voice increases.

The salesman, the lawyer, the doctor, the teacher, even the minister will find it relatively easy to use his voice adequately in spite of a bad cold. The actor's position is more precarious. But with voice training of sufficiently high caliber he may be able to go through his performance even though handicapped by a respiratory infection.

Among those who make professional use of their voice, the singer, above all, must practice intelligent hygiene. Without good general health and intactness of all vocal organs, execution of his art is impossible. This knowledge, unfortunately, often leads to a preoccupation with the health of his voice which is dangerous in itself. Finding the proper middle course between sensible precautions and dangerous pampering is difficult and requires a lot of common sense.

In this chapter we are dealing with the problems of preserving health and preventing disease, with special emphasis on perfect functioning of the vocal organs. Since the speaking and singing voice can be put to a great variety of uses, no one simple set of rules can be laid down regarding intelligent hygiene. While ordinary precaution may be sufficient in many instances, a regime affecting all phases of daily life may be necessary in others.

We shall refer to the singer rather frequently, inasmuch as his profession requires the highest degree of specialization in the use of the voice. He stands to gain the most by following a strict program of daily hygiene. If you belong to one of the less sensitive groups, we trust that you will take our advice with a grain of salt.

To a large extent, preservation of health means prevention of disease. One of the reasons for the vulnerability of the vocal organs lies in the fact that, by an unhappy coincidence, they form one of the frontiers on which the daily battle against disease is fought. In a way, the whole respiratory tract—nose, mouth, larynx, windpipe, bronchi—belongs to the surface of the body. It forms an extension of the surface into the depth, like the pockets of our suits. While our skin is reasonably tough and not easily penetrated by invading germs and viruses, the mucous membranes which line all vocal organs are delicate and vulnerable.

On the subject of vocal hygiene our modern textbooks teach hardly any more than do the chapters written in the days of antiquity. Quintilian, the Roman rethor and author of *De Institutione Oratorica*, the first work on the art of public speaking, advises his readers to lead a simple life, eat sensibly and to get plenty of rest and sleep, a recommendation that need hardly be improved upon. Even lozenges, gargles, medicated fluids, licorice and turpentine, so popular with singers and speakers in this age of patent medicines, were already used by Athenian rethors and Roman actors.

During the Middle Ages, denial of bodily needs and comforts was regarded as a virtue, and in the field of vocal hygiene those days were dark ones too. Since the beginning of the Renaissance, however, with the singer and speaker gaining increasing public prominence countless volumes have been written on the proper care of the voice.

It is therefore with some humility that we approach the task of discussing vocal hygiene. The best way to begin might be to consider the influence of the conditions which rule our daily lives. The most outstanding of these are probably *weather* and *climate*. By weather, we mean the daily changes and fluctuations of atmospheric conditions, while climate applies to the average weather in a given locale. Both weather and climate act primarily upon the surface of our body, the outer surface of the skin and the hidden surface of the mucous membranes.

Among the mammals which require a stable body temperature for the maintenance of life, we humans are the species which relies most heavily on the skin as a regulator of body temperature. Exposed to high temperatures, our skin gives off body heat by perspiring, while in cold weather it helps preserve warmth through the constricting action of the fine blood capillaries. The vocal organs, too, are part of this balancing mechanism. As we have seen in Chapter II, our nose brings inhaled air to the degree of temperature and humidity which the mucous membranes of the deeper respiratory tract require for good health.

With few exceptions, our North American climate is characterized by strong variations in temperature and humidity. It is somewhat paradoxical that the weather we like least is best for our vocal organs and vice versa. On muggy days the air we inhale is warm and saturated with moisture, almost ideal for our mucous membranes. During a summer heat wave, of course, the boon to respiration is more than offset by the languishing effect of the weather on the body as a whole. But the nice crisp winter days with bright skies and invigorating winds are the dangerous ones. The incidence of respiratory infections reaches its peak not during the rainy periods when everyone complains about the weather, but during the cold spells when we are in high spirits and little inclined to worry about it. Then our nose finds it hard to keep up with the need for air conditioning and our skin is chilled by icy winds. It is in such weather that our mucous membranes deserve special consideration. When we leave the house and walk along the street on a cold day carrying on a conversation we are exposing our throat and vocal cords to the rigors of chilly dry air and depriving our mucous membranes of the warmth and moisture which only nose breathing can provide.

If you are in good physical condition, your body will not find it too difficult to adjust to the daily changes of the weather. The teacher, the lawyer and the minister who work in the same place all year round do not ordinarily need to worry so much about the effect of atmospheric conditions on their vocal organs. The artist, the lecturer, on the other hand, are faced with a different situation. Modern means of travel enable the actor on the road, the concert singer on tour and the lecturer whose itinerary calls for appearances in a different city every night to move from one climatic zone to another quickly and abruptly.

The ease with which we can cross the continent or even circle the earth by plane makes us forget the fact that our body is called upon to make tremendous adjustments. Our heart, blood vessels, lungs, skin and mucous membranes are all sorely taxed while we are carried, within just a few hours, from the seacoast to the mountains, from temperate zones to the tropics.

An artist who travels frequently has to be in good physical condition to stand the strain of such sudden adaptations. And even then he should, if at all possible, arrange his schedule to include a day of acclimatization before an appearance. If you have ever flown from the East Coast to Denver, for example, you will remember how dry and papery your throat felt after a few hours in the thin mountain air, how your heart beat faster and your breathing was accelerated. In such a state, satisfactory voice performance is very difficult. Even intonation may suffer at high altitudes until the fine muscles which control the vocal cords have become adjusted to the low density of the air.

A horse, brought up from the plains to the mountains, refuses to canter until it has become acclimated. Human lungs, hearts and mucous membranes are entitled to the same consideration.

Of course, man has one big advantage over animals. We have learned to wear *clothing* as protection against the vicissitudes of the weather. The only trouble is that, to a large extent, clothing has lost its original purpose. It has become a symbol of social standing, a playground for constantly changing fashions and has spoiled our natural powers of body resistance. From a strictly medical viewpoint, women often wear too little clothing and men too much. Women dress very sensibly in warm weather, but how they manage to brave winter days in cobweb stockings, open shoes and hardly any underwear is a secret which a doctor cannot hope to understand. Men, on the other hand, insist on wearing numerous layers of clothing, shirts with closed collars, strangling neckties and tight belts. But we do not expect to conquer the tyranny of fashion and convention by printed advice and therefore shall limit ourselves to a few remarks about the importance of proper clothing in the care of the vocal organs.

Apart from moral, esthetic and social considerations clothing has just one function: to form an insulating layer of air, under fabric, around the body. More harm is done by too many and too heavy clothes than by too few and too light ones. On the whole, the healthy skin makes all the necessary adjustments with great speed, and light clothing keeps it in good condition. Dressing heavily to avoid colds has quite frequently the opposite effect.

One of our habitual cold patients is a middle-aged singer who comes to our office swaddled in every conceivable kind of garment. Watching him get undressed for a chest examination is to witness a major production: having shed several mufflers, a heavy suit, vest and sweater, he finally emerges in long woolen underwear quite suitable for a Canadian fur trapper which he does not shed until the first summer heat wave. In winter and summer, his skin lives in a permanent Turkish bath. Exhausted by so much sweating, it has long ceased to function as the body's main line of defense and the result is a patient with an almost uninterrupted series of upper respiratory infections.

The case just cited may be an extreme one, but all too many singers still pamper their body by dressing too warmly. The younger generation is getting to be more sensible; the modern trend toward light, informal clothes is definitely a boon to preservation of health and prevention of colds.

Proper *heating* of our homes is another important factor in maintaining health. A good heating system should provide just enough warmth to make us feel comfortable, keep our heads cool and our feet warm and, at the same time, stabilize the humidity at a favorable level. Unfortunately, conventional steam heating meets none of these requirements. American homes, offices and community buildings are notoriously overheated; the floors are the coldest part of our rooms, and the already dry winter air is further desiccated by the hot radiators. European visitors keep asking us how we can stand it. The answer should be, we cannot.

Every fall, the beginning of the heating season brings to our offices singers, actors and others who use their voices professionally, all complaining of dryness of the throat. Since we cannot change the heating system, the only way out is artificial humidification. This is easier said than done, however, for even when all windows and doors are closed the air in a room is constantly changing. To keep it from becoming overly dry, moisture has to be added all the time. Most every medical supply house now carries relatively inexpensive humidifiers which will bring relief to those suffering from dryness of the mucous membranes in the nose, throat and larynx. In apartments and houses where the bedroom adjoins the bathroom, a humidifier can be improvised by leaving the door open and letting the hot shower run for a while.

Let us now consider the problem of *ventilation.* To open or not to open the windows is an unresolved controversy between the advocates of tough living on one side and the enemies of draft on the other. Being inclined to sympathize with the fresh-air fans, we would like to report that, from a medical point of view, they are better equipped in the fight against colds. Actually, large-scale statistical research has shown no appreciable difference in the incidence of colds among those who sleep with windows open and those who do not.

The rule of common sense applies to ventilation just as it applies to the other subjects brought up in this discussion. There is a healthy medium between the singer who is forever concerned lest he catch a breath of cool air and the advocate of rigorous living who refuses to close the window in any weather. In the daytime when we are on the move, a healthy body can well endure a lot of fresh air; but when we are asleep, all body functions slow down and our skin and mucous membranes fare best when the temperature of the surrounding air is comfortable and even.

In the realm of personal habits, *nutrition* is one area in which the most serious offenses are committed. In this age of preoccupation with diets, almost everyone knows exactly what foods he ought to eat and, it would appear, avoids them conscientiously. All of us are forever overeating after having carefully selected the wrong things. We prefer the whitest of breads, the richest desserts and have come to believe that meat is the most important food.

There does not seem to be much sense in repeating what you can read in almost every magazine, namely, that our diet should be well planned with a strong accent on fresh vegetables, salads, fruit, whole-grain bread and dairy products. Everybody knows that anyhow. The spirit is strong but the sweet tooth is our weakness. Let us only point out that the mucous membranes prefer a diet in which starches are limited to a minimum. This is especially important in those cases in which an overproduction of phlegm interferes with free nasal breathing and clarity of the voice. Experiments with children have proven the value of low carbohydrate diet under such circumstances.

Overindulgence in starches is, of course, mainly responsible for making us a nation with a tendency to overweight. Conversely, public taste demands that the artists who appear in opera, theater, motion pictures and on television be slim-waisted. The fat singer is a thing of the past. As a result, countless performers are forever struggling to keep their weight down to a minimum, frequently to the detriment of general and vocal health.

Everyone has an optimum weight which best suits his body structure. Generally speaking, that weight is somewhat less than what most men over forty actually weigh, and somewhat more than what women of all ages consider desirable. Rather than alternating between sporadic spells of fast reducing when the newest nine-day-wonder diet appears in your favorite newspaper and subsequent flings of overeating, it is far wiser to maintain one's body weight at the level which experience has shown to be most conducive to the maintenance of well-being, vigor and resistance.

Just a word about the timing of meals. Almost everyone who performs in public instinctively avoids eating a heavy meal before an appearance. Afterward, however, there is the temptation to eat too much. The release of tensions after a performance brings with it proverbial hunger and thirst which easily lead to overindulgence in food and drink at very late hours. Poor sleep and overweight are usually the result.

We all have become very *vitamin* conscious in recent years and help support a gigantic industry that produces the multicolored capsules which we take to atone for all dietary transgressions. Actually, a well-planned diet contains all necessary vitamins in sufficient amounts. If you eat properly you should not need vitamin pills.

Still, we cannot deny that a surprisingly large number of patients—rich as well as poor—are borderline cases of vitamin deficiency. Many of these deficiencies manifest themselves in the mucous membranes of the respiratory tract. We find it, therefore, quite important to watch the professional vocalist for possible signs of vitamin shortage.

In taking vitamins, one fact must be kept in mind: the body does not store vitamins but accepts them only in such amounts as are needed at a given time. In other words, if you buy and take vitamins with which your body is already amply supplied you are throwing your money away. Only your doctor can tell you whether your vitamin level needs boosting.

Ask him to recommend a reliable brand which fills your temporary needs. Do not shop around for bargains. An inexpensive brand might well be useless because the amount of vitamins is too small, because prolonged storage has led to deterioration in the capsule or, worse, but unfortunately not infrequent, because an irresponsible manufacturer has misstated the actual contents.

It is with some hesitation that we approach our next subject —the use of nicotine and alcohol. The pressure of social convention and personal habits, the weight of philosophical and even religious convictions make it difficult to pass dispassionate judgment. We propose to limit our discussion to an evaluation of both substances as they affect the vocal organs.

We might as well confess right away that we smoke moderately ourselves—no smoker will admit to more—and enjoy a drink in good company. Having admitted that much, perhaps our opinion will carry more weight when we state categorically that nicotine and alcohol (at least as a habit) are the avowed enemies of the speaker and singer.

The case against *nicotine* is simple. We are not concerned here with its effect on the heart and the blood vessels but with the direct irritation of the mucous membranes caused by the inhaled smoke. In this respect, pipe and cigar smoking is less harmful since deep inhalation is rarely practiced by its addicts. The cigarette smoker who brings the smoke down to the vocal cords, windpipe and even bronchi is the real sufferer.

Whenever we want to demonstrate the effect of smoking to a recalcitrant patient we show him a little experiment which you can easily perform for your own enlightenment. Blow cigarette smoke into a highball glass, cover the glass with a sheet of white paper, turn it upside down and let it stand for a few minutes. When you remove the glass, you will see a distinct yellow circle—it shows up better in daylight—and you will realize the extent of irritation of your mucous membranes by the continuous deposits of coal tars from the smoke.

If that does not scare you properly nothing we could cite here will. But we should like to state, as a concluding remark, that there exists more than a suspicion that the recent rise in the incidence of lung cancer is related to the increase of excessive smoking in all groups of the population.

The case against *alcohol* cannot be stated quite so easily. For thousands of years, alcohol has been used because of its stimulating or rather inhibition-loosening effect on the brain. If taken before a performance to overcome the tensions of stage fright, its blessings are questionable. Alcohol interferes with judgment, substituting a delusive satisfaction for real mastery of performance, and it impairs muscular co-ordination and physical efficiency to an extent which might well be detrimental to the speaker or singer. Besides, alcohol dilates the blood capillaries and thus causes an increased production of mucus—an added undesirable effect on the vocal organs.

Habitual use of alcohol is definitely harmful to the voice as the rough hoarseness of the "whiskey tenor" will attest. Finally, alcohol upsets the delicate heat balance of the body. It gives our skin a deceptive feeling of warmth, while we are losing heat at a rapid rate. Such chilling makes the body more vulnerable to colds.

As long as you limit your consumption of alcohol to an occasional drink following a performance and avoid exposure to cold weather afterward, no harm is done. But before a performance, leave alcohol to the members of your audience who might thus get into the proper frame of mind for a gracious reception of your artistry.

By now you are undoubtedly tired of being told what *not* to do and having *Verboten* signs plastered all over your personal life. So, for a change, let us turn to the things you *can* and should do.

Rest, for instance. Although we often complain that the mad rush of modern life does not give us sufficient time for rest, we all agree that plenty of sleep at night and refreshing siestas during the day are highly desirable. We dislike intensely to give commonplace advice which is easily pronounced but hard to follow (such as the doctor's famous stand-by, "take it easy for a while"). The competitive struggle for success in arts and professions usually leaves most of us little latitude in shaping personal habits. Yet it must be said that a fair amount of undisturbed sleep is essential to the maintenance of good general health and for proper functioning and resilience of the vocal organs. In this connection, the group to whom this book is dedicated is often confronted with a special problem: how to get the necessary rest period before a vocal performance. The curse of the traveling lecturer and the actor and singer on the road is the pressure of social obligations. Having spent a restless night in a sleeping car, he is often asked to accept well-meant invitations to luncheons, teas and receptions. Even at the risk of incurring the displeasure of hostesses and agents, it is far wiser to decline such voice-straining engagements politely and to rest up for the evening's performance instead.

How valuable is *exercise*? With certain reservations, regular moderate exercise is healthy and can be heartily endorsed. By moderate, we mean not only the amount of exercise, but also the spirit in which it is undertaken. Voice professionals of all types work under considerable nervous strain. Sports should help them to relax and take their mind off their worries. Competitive games only add new tensions. We can learn a lesson from the protagonists of real sportsmanship, the old Greeks and the English who have never forgotten that sport is basically play. The often heard expression "to play hard" is a contradiction in itself. If you cannot restrain yourself from comparing scores constantly, you had better stay home and rest with a good book.

If you are middle-aged and not accustomed to regular exercise do not decide that now is the time to recapture your youthful figure through strenuous athletics. The consequences might be disastrous.

Swimming is an ideal sport for the vocalist. It stimulates

the skin, encourages deep breathing and smooth muscle action. Walking is one of the best and most neglected forms of exercise. From a medical point of view, the value of golf lies mainly in the fact that it induces people to walk a couple of miles. Running at a comfortable trot is excellent for younger people, since it improves control and economy of breathing. Many gymnasiums have tracks for the purpose, but a quiet country road is even better.

Whatever form of exercise you prefer, do it at a leisurely pace, forget about scores and, above all, enjoy yourself.

Our next subject is of particular interest to women: the influence of menstruation and pregnancy on the vocal organs.

Regarding *menstruation* it might be worth noting here that European opera companies have a special clause in their contracts which permits female singers to excuse themselves from all performances during the menstrual period. Schedules are filed with the management and plans made accordingly. In the United States, on the other hand, artists are expected and do perform without regard to menstruation.

What are the medical facts? Ever since the famous English throat specialist Morel Mackenzie—who, by the way, wrote in 1888 the first scientific book on the hygiene of the vocal organs, that is still a classic—published his observations on the connection between the female reproductive organs and the nasal turbinates, we have known that many women suffer from nasal congestion immediately before and at the beginning of their menstrual period. We have furthermore learned to regard the whole respiratory tract as a unit that is sensitive to changes in the hormonal balance. Many women experience no discomfort in the nose or lower respiratory tract during menstruation but others do in varying degrees. Besides, a number of women complain of other circulatory upsets during those days, of abdominal discomfort that interferes with free breathing, and of depressive moods.

As a general rule, singing or acting during menstruation will

have no harmful effects as long as the artist does not try to overcome any indisposition by force. Here again, superior technique is the surest compensation for any temporary impairment of perfect vocal function. Do not expect to be at your best during the menstrual period; avoid, if possible, important engagements which produce additional tensions, and rely on your technique. But do not use any force which might harm your voice.

Pregnancy does not interfere with voice performance during the first five or six months. Some women are able to sing freely and without effort up to an advanced stage of pregnancy. Generally, however, it is best to give up professional singing and acting during the last months. Not only may hormonal influences on the mucous membranes become more pronounced by that time, but the growth of the baby will interfere with abdominal breathing.

After delivery, the overstretched abdominal muscles slowly return to their normal state. In view of the importance of abdominal breathing and muscular control for vocal quality, special care must be taken to strengthen the abdominal muscles. Breathing exercises should be resumed very soon, followed by active muscular training and moderate vocalization. Of course, nothing should be done before the obstetrician gives the green light.

Allergy of any marked degree constitutes a handicap for the speaker or singer and requires care and treatment. The majority of all allergies are due to substances we inhale—like pollen, dust, animal hair, molds—and produce respiratory symptoms such as congestion of the nose, sneezing, running discharge, itching of the throat, cough, wheezing from the chest. At the peak of an allergic attack or during a seasonal bout, as with hay fever, the normal functioning of the vocal organs is impaired, sometimes to the extent of total professional disability.

Seasonably limited allergies are bad enough. Ragweed hay

fever, for instance (from which about three and a half million people suffer in the United States), lasts until the end of September and makes the opening of the music and theatrical season pure torment for many artists. Dust and other year-round allergies are even worse, in that they are constantly interfering with professional activities. Above all, the untreated allergy may lead to asthmatic symptoms, one of the severest handicaps under which a speaker or vocal artist can labor.

For these reasons, *treatment* of an allergy is part of vocal hygiene. Limitations of space forbid going into details. You will need the help of a doctor anyhow with special experience in testing and treating allergic conditions. Suffice it to say that allergies—once determined by conclusive tests—can be dealt with in three ways: by eliminating the offending agents, by building up resistance through so-called desensitization, or by the use of the new antihistaminic drugs.

Elimination of the offending agent is possible in cases of food allergies by excluding such foods from the diet. To a lesser extent it is feasible with animal hair and dust: household pets can be banished and pillows and mattresses protected with dustproof covers. Air conditioning affords temporary relief, but the patient feels worse than before if he has to leave the comfort of filtered air.

The *antihistaminics* of which dozens of brands are now available do *not* cure allergy. They only suppress symptoms. They are valuable in providing fast temporary relief, but they do not create any resistance to allergy. Besides, these drugs produce unwanted secondary effects in a large percentage of patients, such as drowsiness which interferes with the presence of mind, reliability of memory and muscular co-ordination so important to the speaker, actor and singer. Furthermore, the purely symptomatic action of antihistaminic drugs gives no protection against the danger of developing asthmatic troubles.

In attempting to control allergies our best bet is still *desensi-*

tization—the gradual building up of resistance by injections of allergen extracts of increasing strength. This method produces excellent results in cases of pollen and dust allergies, especially if combined with occasional small doses of antihistaminics on peak days of exposure. Up to 80 per cent of the patients suffering from these types of allergies can be made symptom-free or, at least, quite comfortable.

Treatment of allergy is one aspect of vocal hygiene which definitely calls for the help of a doctor. Competent medical supervision may mean the difference between an insurmountable handicap in the professional use of the voice and a wide margin of safety and freedom from discomfort.

From birth until death, our voice reflects the various stages of physical development through which we pass. The first cry of the baby, the child's high-pitched voice, the changing voice of the adolescent, all play an important part toward the final shaping of the adult speaking and singing voice. We shall discuss this in the next chapter.

Very little is known about the influence of advanced *age* on the vocal organs. This is particularly regrettable when we consider that with rising life expectancy the number of people of sixty is on the increase and includes many who use their voice professionally such as teachers, ministers, lawyers and even singers.

Geriatrics, the science dealing with the diseases of the aged, has become a new field in medicine. Geriatrics of the voice is a field of research which should attract the interest of all those who specialize in speech and voice therapy. Study of the effects of hormonal, vitamin, drug and exercise therapy on the aging voice may result in a more active approach to the problem.

Until such time, we must restrict ourselves to describing the effects of advancing age on the voice: the joints between the cartilages of the larynx move less smoothly, the cartilages themselves become more rigid, muscle co-ordination is impaired and muscular strength weakened. This results in loss of vocal power, uncertainty of intonation and the typical tremolo and wavering we associate with old people's voices. Changes in the hormonal balance may cause inversion of the sex characteristics—the male voice becoming higher and the female voice assuming a masculine timbre. As with all the other bodily changes which accompany old age wide individual differences exist with regard to the rapidity and intensity of such changes. Constitutional and hereditary factors have a determining influence, and it is at this point also that the long-term effects of well-regulated life make themselves felt.

The professional speaker will find it much easier to adjust to advancing age than the singer who may feel the negative effects much sooner. It was indeed an unforgettable experience to have heard the great Mattia Battistini sing Don Giovanni at the age of seventy. But many others age prematurely, in body as well as in voice. Those with poor vocal technique are the first to fall by the wayside, while the singer who has devoted a lifetime to perfecting his technique and preserving his health intelligently may be able to lead an active professional life in spite of advancing years; but there are no set rules.

It is indeed hard for the artist who is young in spirit and rich in accumulated experience to accept the inevitability of age. One of the saddest aspects of a voice doctor's practice is to witness the decline of a great voice after the age of sixty and to have to watch the hopeless struggle of many an artist who tries, often in the face of financial insecurity, to prolong a career which is rapidly coming to an end.

The only thing that may ease this tragic situation is to help the artist face the facts and come to terms with reality before audiences reject his deteriorating performances. Here, as is so frequently the case, the doctor's task is mainly a psychological one; but it is a frustrating experience which makes us hope that future research will equip us to take a more active approach.

This chapter has become rather long, as was to be expected, since we have dealt with a key subject in our field. Eight out of ten questions which are addressed to us after a lecture on voice problems concern the hygiene of everyday living. In concluding we should like to answer the most frequent of all questions: can one prevent colds?

First and foremost, there is no better way of *preventing a cold* than to build up a healthy body. It is impossible to avoid exposure especially in wintertime when most everyone sneezes and coughs at us. But it is possible to increase resistance. A body whose resistance has been undermined by inadequate diet, too much heavy clothing and too little rest and exercise is easily conquered by infection. Therefore, everything we do to build up body strength, resilience and hardiness helps to protect us against respiratory infections.

There is no short cut to good health. You cannot prevent colds by simply taking a few tablets or cold shots. The common cold is a virus infection which produces only a short-lived immunity. As yet there exists no effective vaccine.

The so-called *cold shots* try a kind of detour approach. Most of the complications of colds are caused not by the original cold virus but by various germs which invade the body after the cold virus has attacked it. The purpose of cold vaccines is to build up an immunity to these germs. Although some patients claim to be benefited by such shots, the results are rather questionable. Statistics show no appreciable difference in the frequency and duration of colds among those who have been treated with cold shots and those who have not. We personally do not recommend them and give the shots only if a patient insists on them.

Oral cold vaccines—taken by mouth in tablet or capsule form—have, so far, produced very unsatisfactory results. All research workers who have tested them on large groups agree in rejecting these vaccines.

The only type of vaccination that has proven at all effective is the use of *influenza shots*. The influenza vaccine which the Army successfully tested during the war is easy to take: one full or, better yet, two half doses given at the beginning of the winter, followed by booster shots after three months. The vaccine, however, affords protection only against the most common strains of influenza virus. Still, its use can be endorsed as a harmless method of building up resistance against one of the most debilitating respiratory infections.

Several years ago, antihistaminic *cold tablets* were introduced with loud fanfares by press and advertising and tremendous sales to a hopeful public. Since then, the medical profession has had the opportunity to evaluate these drugs, and, just as the experts predicted, the results are disappointing indeed. Colds are infections. Antihistaminics, as we have pointed out, are drugs that suppress allergic symptoms. They can hardly be expected to cure or prevent colds. A large group of college students was subjected to an experiment to determine the effectiveness of cold tablets. Half of the students were given genuine cold tablets, the other half sugar pills which were similar in appearance. The incidence of colds was found to be the same in both groups.

As we have said in the beginning, when it comes to hygiene of the vocal organs, the advice of old Quintilian and the teachers of Italian Bel Canto is hard to beat: keep your body in good shape to withstand the rigors of wind and weather; dress sensibly but do not undermine your resistance by pampering yourself; plan your meals in accordance with nutritional requirements; get as much rest and sleep as possible; exercise moderately.

Finding the proper middle course between the two equally dangerous extremes of willfully neglecting the body and oversolicitous pampering is the most important maxim in vocal hygiene. So long as the body and the vocal organs are accustomed to a healthy routine an occasional fling will do no harm. As in all others areas of life, common sense is what matters.

VIII. *Self-treatment of Colds*

SOONER OR LATER, EVERYBODY GETS A COLD. SOME OF US MIGHT be lucky and escape colds for a while because of high personal resistance or lack of infecting contacts. The average person keeps getting colds with depressing regularity, at least twice a year. Colds, as has been said very often, are inescapable as weather, death and taxes.

Contrary to popular opinion, not even the climate you live in makes much difference. If you do not rely on the claims of Chambers of Commerce but on "cold" statistics you will find almost the same rate of infection in Florida, the Midwest, California or Alaska.

This is as it should be because the common cold is first and foremost an *infection*. As a rule, people are strangely reluctant to accept this fact. Their attitude is a classical example of the influence of a semantic error on our thinking. The term "cold" has stressed the part played by chilling in contracting a cold to the degree that the importance of infection is always underrated. Consequently people with colds feel often compelled to search for some "mistake" they must have made.

Mumps or measles are accepted as unavoidable accidents because we know that infection can hit us when we expect it least. But we react to our colds as if we had committed a sin. We search our conscience for the window we forgot to close, the muffler we left behind, the rubbers we should have worn.

True, chilling plays its part in the mechanism of getting a cold but it is not the decisive factor. You may become the victim of a cold without any chilling, but *never* without an infection with the virus of the common cold.

We hear a lot about *viruses* these days. What used to be an interesting research problem known only to bacteriologists has become a household word in the last ten years. "Virus infection" is now a convenient label for all kinds of fevers of unknown origin and a favorite diagnosis with the patient who likes a fancy label for his sickness.

Viruses are different from the ordinary run of germs in a number of negative ways: they cannot be seen under the microscope (except as bare shadows with tremendous electronic enlargement), they cannot be separated from any fluid that contains them even by the finest filters, and they cannot be isolated and cultured by the usual laboratory methods.

The list of infectious diseases that are caused by viruses is very long with new additions extending it constantly. Measles, German measles, mumps, polio, influenza, smallpox, to mention only a few, are virus infections.

The *virus of the common cold* beats them all in omnipresence and frequency of infections. The cold virus is unique in that it acts as the door-opener for many bacterial infections. The virus attacks first, weakens the resistance of the mucous membranes which then may be invaded by germs—like streptococci, staphylococci, pneumococci—that lurk everywhere. If they take over, all kinds of complications may develop, such as ear infections, sinusitis, tonsillitis, laryngitis, bronchitis, pneumonia.

The common cold, if it remains limited to the primary cold virus infection, is a relatively harmless, self-limited disease. Its significance and importance lies in the possibility of secondary bacterial infection.

Most virus infections leave in their wake a long lasting immunity, some—like measles or polio—for life, others for years. But the cold virus can hit us again after a few weeks. It has not yet been isolated, and no vaccine is available that could protect us. Considering the amount of misery that colds cause to mankind, directly or in the form of complications, they are the biggest enemy to public health and would deserve more attention than they get in medical research.

Chilling diminishes the resistance of our mucous membranes to infection. It has to be rather protracted to lower the temperature of the nasal surfaces by contraction of the small blood vessels. The draft from an open window, the blast of the wind at the street corner are, as a rule, offset by the ability of our body to make fast adjustments to changes in temperature.

We get a cold because somebody gives it to us and because our resistance to infection has dropped to a low level. We call for the police if a pickpocket tries to steal our purse, but we tolerate with indifference the thief of our health who spreads infection by sneezing and coughing in public places and conveyances without bothering to use his hand as a cover. We look at every open window with fear but we weaken our body resistance by lack of sleep, poor eating habits and the hectic rush of modern life.

There is no need to describe the symptoms of a cold. We all know them from frequent experience. While to the average person an uncomplicated cold is just a nuisance to be borne with more or less grace it is the terror of the man or woman who uses his voice professionally. To him, colds constitute an ever present occupational hazard. The battlefield of the cold and of its complications are the vocal organs. The cold impairs their function, usually at the most inopportune moments. The cold leads the list of the pet hates of the singer, actor or speaker, even ahead of critics, producers or unreceptive audiences.

Unfortunately, no specific therapy exists against the common cold. As long as no drug that attacks the virus of the cold is available, the defense against the invader is left to the powers of resistance of the body. The only sensible treatment of colds consists of making it easier for the body to concentrate on the job of fighting the infection by relieving it, as much as possible, from other work. In other words, taking the cold seriously, staying at home or even better in bed for a day or two.

But that goes against human nature (and we doctors who should know better are as bad as the rest). We all talk about our colds, we annoy our families by complaining about our misery, we want to be pitied as a patient, but we refuse to behave like one. We keep on running around, spreading infection right and left, and, instead of giving our body a fair chance, we "treat" our cold with our favorite remedies.

For, in treating colds, everybody is an expert. There is no other field in medicine, where superstitions, time-honored misconceptions, short-lived fads are so widely practiced and hotly defended as in dealing with a cold.

One of the oldest favorites with cold patients—particularly if they are men—is *alcohol.* People are seldom at loss for an excuse to take a drink, but in the case of an approaching cold the belief in the germ-killing abilities of alcohol gives a special medical dignity to the consumption of a few drinks.

Actually, alcohol fights infection only if rubbed on the skin. Taken internally it upsets the heat balance of the body. It dilates the blood vessels and gives us a deceptive feeling of warmth. The skin loses heat rapidly while we feel comfortable.

The patient who takes a drink to fight the chilliness of the first stage of a cold and then proceeds with his daily chores creates only more favorable conditions for an intense chilling without becoming aware of it. He should wait until he can go home and intends to stay there. Then a drink will help to return body comfort. But no amount of alcohol will disturb the cold virus in its temporary conquest of our body. We do not want to keep you from the enjoyment of your favorite drink, but you cannot expect our medical blessing for your personal habits.

If you begin to sneeze, your first reflex is probably to open the drawer or the medicine chest where you keep your favorite brand of tablets for just this emergency. Thanks to a tremendous effort of advertising, *aspirin* is your most likely choice. Again we have to disappoint you by saying that aspirin has no direct effect whatsoever on the cold virus. Aspirin is a trade name for acetylsalicylic acid. It belongs to the family of the so-called antipyretics. They inhibit the heat regulating centers of the brain and lower body temperatures by perspiration to a certain degree.

Now, increase in temperature is one of the devices of the body to fight infection. To bring the temperature of the blood down makes us feel more comfortable but, at the same time, counteracts the self-help of nature.

Aspirin and related drugs, like phenacetin, have their place in medicine as mild pain killers. Some of the complications of the common cold create pain. Aspirin or similar drugs are then helpful to take the edge off the discomfort until the infection is conquered. But in the fight against a cold, aspirin is without value, and the almost mystic reputation of the drug as a cold remedy has no basis.

A few years ago, the antihistaminics were introduced with great publicity as *cold tablets*. In the meantime sober evaluation has reduced the exaggerated claims to a minimum. Antihistaminics, as we have seen in the last chapter, are drugs that suppress allergic symptoms. Colds are infections. The best that can be expected from these cold tablets is a suppression of some of the symptoms of a cold in patients with allergic tendencies. On the other hand, the antihistaminics create drowsiness in many patients; they impair the speed of muscular reaction which makes driving a car while taking these tablets a risky business; and they can be dangerous to small children.

If we cannot fight cold actively, we can, at least, try to alleviate the symptoms as much as possible. Of these, the stuffiness of the nose and the profuse nasal discharge are particularly unpleasant. For relief of nasal blockage nose drops are widely used.

The ideal *nose drops* should contain a *vasoconstrictor*, one of the drugs which make the nasal membranes shrink by contraction of the small blood vessels; they should be *isotonic*, meaning equal in concentration to the body fluids; and they should be slightly *alkaline*.

The most widely used vasoconstrictor is *ephedrine* which in a 1 per cent solution produces a mild shrinking of the mucous membranes. A number of similarly effective vasoconstrictors are marketed under brand names. They all use a watery basis of isotonic concentration. The simplest isotonic diluent is saline, a .9 per cent solution of salt in distilled water which equals the concentration of salt in the body fluids.

Alkalinity of nose drops is desirable because the important self-cleaning mechanism of the mucous membranes by ciliary action (see Chapter III) depends on the slight alkalinity of the nasal mucus. In colds and other infections the nose becomes slightly acid which results in a slowing down or stopping of ciliary movement. In a classical series of investigations, Dr. Fabricant has shown that slightly alkaline medication helps to restore normal ciliary function. The 1 per cent solution of ephedrine in saline fulfills this need.

Nose drops of high concentration or of acid p^H (the chemical measurement for acidity or alkalinity) should not be used. For this reason the protein-silver compounds which were the medical vogue for a while are definitely not recommended.

The best way to administer nose drops is to instill them with a dropper into the nostrils while lying on the back with the head extended as far back as possible. A small pillow under the neck makes it easier to assume this position. Another, equally effective position is to lie on one side and to let the drops fall into the lower nostril; then to turn around and to repeat the process with the other nostril.

Nose drops should be used sparingly, three to four drops into each nostril at a time and at no shorter intervals than three hours. Overdosage irritates the mucous membranes and might raise the blood pressure in sensitive persons. Small children should not be given any nose drops without the advice of a doctor.

A more effective way of administering nose drops is in the form of *sprays*. The small atomizers which can be bought in any drug store have a number of advantages. They produce a fine spray that covers a larger surface than the drops with a minimum of the drug. They can be used in the sitting position, and they are easily sterilized.

The latter is particularly important because the conventional dropper, once it has touched the nose will contaminate the contents of the bottle. Bottles with nose droppers should *never* be used again for another cold. The contents are almost invariably polluted with hosts of germs.

Even if it hurts you, throw your nose drops into the garbage can when your cold is gone. The half-filled bottle you like to save for future use will cost you dearly by giving you or your family "nose dropper disease" a few months later.

Oily nose drops, a great favorite of past years with patients and doctors, are definitely out. The paraffin that forms the base of most of these drops glides easily from the throat into the windpipe and from there into the lungs. It has been shown that prolonged use of oily nose drops may produce quite nasty inflammatory changes in the lung tissues.

To sum up: use 1 per cent ephedrine solution in saline or the brand-equivalent of it (your doctor will be glad to recommend you his preference); use it sparingly; keep in mind that nose drops or sprays should make you more comfortable without interfering with the mechanism by which the body gets rid of a cold. A certain amount of congestion of the mucous membranes and of nasal discharge is quite desirable. It brings the healing forces of the blood into the infected area and helps to throw off the invading germs and the debris of the battle. Overdosage of vasoconstrictors will only prolong the normal course of a cold.

Modern medicine has opened so many new avenues for active approach in the treatment of diseases that we have, somehow, lost sight of the fact that the main burden in conquering infection will always be with our body. Give it rest from all unnecessary work and it will expel the cold virus within a few days. The professional of the speaking or singing voice stands more to lose by the complications of colds that are the inevitable result of running around with an infection. Ounces of nose drops and bottles of tablets will not do for you what one day in the equalizing warmth of your bed can achieve.

Local heat is one of the oldest remedies for all kinds of local aches. To expose an infected part of our body to any form of local heat means to create hyperemia, an increased flood of healing blood through the dilated blood vessels of skin or deeper tissues. The short-wave or diathermy machines which lend so much glamour to the doctor's office are needed where deeper parts of the body have to be reached by radiating heat.

To get heat to the mucous membranes of nose and throat, the old-fashioned *inhalation of steam* serves just as well. If you use it at home you have to keep in mind two points.

The dilation of blood vessels which is the immediate consequence of the application of local heat might increase the discomfort in your already congested nose. If that happens you are better off without it.

Do not inhale steam if you have to leave the house shortly afterward. During a cold the mucous membranes have temporarily lost their ability to make quick adjustments to changes in temperature. To wake up in the morning with a cold, swallow a couple of aspirins, inhale steam for five minutes, dry your face while you gulp your coffee and then rush out to work means to court disaster. The aspirin will make you perspire, thereby cooling the skin, the overheated mucous membranes will be chilled by the cold outside air and the germs that lie in wait will have a field day. You will return in the evening with the makings of a fine sinusitis, laryngitis or even bronchitis.

So far, we have spoken only of the nose in a cold. The professional speaker or singer will worry almost as much or even more about his throat. Many colds begin anyhow with a tickling or burning sensation in the upper part of the throat. Too many professionals have the habit of constantly "treating" their throat with all kinds of medication, by way of gargles, lozenges, troches. In times of colds they redouble their efforts in the mistaken belief that they can kill the infection by such measures.

If we doctors want our hands reasonably clean we scrub them with hard brushes and disinfecting soap for a long time. Even then we distrust their sterility and put on rubber gloves for surgical work. If we want to sterilize instruments, which cannot be boiled, we put them into sharp disinfectants for at least half an hour.

The throat would never tolerate such high concentrations. The disinfectants in gargles must be extremely diluted to suit our mucous membranes. Gargling brings them in contact with the throat for a few seconds. How can one expect any germ-killing effect from so short and so weak a contact? The only good that can come from gargling is a superficial kind of cleaning. If the gargle is at least hot it helps to attract the blood into the irritated throat and to stimulate a soothing flow of mucus.

Hot milk, with or without honey, achieves just the same. Whether you apply local heat by steam, hot gargles or any hot drinks it is always the temporary hyperemia that relieves your throat, not the effect of any drugs or special foods you may add to them. The drinking of raw eggs—an old stand-by with singers, ministers, teachers—can be classified only as self-punishment for past sins against vocal hygiene.

The case for *lozenges* or *troches* rests on a rather doubtful basis too. Lozenge is a French intruder into the English language, reminding us of past centuries when fashionable people who never heard of a toothbrush sucked perfumed pastilles for obvious reasons. Troche is the Greek word for medicated tablets.

The lozenges, troches, coughdrops and similar pastilles that are sold to the public by the millions have little effect on the throat. The drugs they contain are weak and without therapeutic value. The glycerine that forms the base of many lozenges dries the membranes out because of its hydroscopic (water-binding) action. The best that can be said about these pastilles is that they stimulate the flow of saliva by the movements of the tongue.

The constant habit of many singers and speakers of using lozenges whenever the throat feels dry confuses the effect of nervous tensions on the throat with the infectious irritation of the cold. The sucking of a lozenge before a speech or an appearance is a kind of psychotherapeutic self-treatment that is, at least, more harmless than the cigarette or the drink.

Aromatic compounds have been used in all forms for thousands of years. Camphor, menthol, aromatic oils (like eucalyptus, pine needle, turpentine) were already great favorites with Greek actors, Roman rethors, Italian singers, and they are still dear to the hearts of cold-suffering patients. They are soothing to mucous membranes by the creation of a sensation of coolness. In the nose they are irritating and should not be used. In sprays or lozenges for the throat they do no harm and satisfy the desire of the patients for a comforting sickroom odor that gives their troubles a certain distinction.

Lately, troches which contain one of the *antibiotics* (like penicillin, aureomycin, terramycin) have been made available. They should *not* be used without the specific advice of the doctor. These troches have their place in the treatment of localized infections of the mouth and throat. Their indiscriminate use in a normal cold can be quite dangerous. Doctors see now quite often allergic reactions to antibiotic troches that create much more misery than the relatively slight discomfort of the throat they were meant to banish.

Altogether, we have to admit that no active therapy of any kind will influence the short course of a common cold with any degree of efficiency. You might now, with some justification, object to the title of this chapter as a promise that was not kept.

But we have to remind you again that one effective self-treatment of colds exists: rest, rest to the body in its fight against the infection and rest to the vocal organs which cannot stand the double burden of local warfare against the invader and of highly complex function in professional use.

To Voltaire is ascribed the malicious remark that "medicine is the art of entertaining the patient while nature takes care of the healing." As wrong as this witticism might be in many medical emergencies that require energetic action, it serves to remind us that in most diseases it is the body itself which does the actual healing.

Somehow it goes against the grain of our hyperactive Western philosophy of life to deal with an unpleasant situation in a passive way. Even in minor diseases, like a cold, we feel compelled to do something about it.

If you follow Voltaire, your only self-treatment of your next cold should consist of entertaining yourself while nature takes care of the rest. You might watch television, solve a crossword puzzle or read a book—maybe even this one—but otherwise just make it easy for your body to do the healing. Stay home for a day, preferably in bed, eat lightly and keep your bowels open—without resorting to harsh drugs. Blow your nose gently to avoid pressing infected mucus into sinuses or middle ears. Use nose drops sparingly to reduce nasal congestion. If you have a headache take an aspirin, no more than three or four during the day.

With this regime, your cold will soon be over, without requiring the help of a doctor. The sacrifice of a day or two at home will pay good dividends in fast recovery or in avoidance of complications.

A normal common cold should be broken in four to six days. If, in spite of reasonable precautions, no improvement of the condition should be observed within this time limit it will be necessary to ask for the help of a doctor.

Other complications that require medical advice are:

The development of a *laryngitis.* This frequent and usually harmless sequel of a cold is, of course, a great handicap for the speaker and singer and requires special treatment;

Severe *headaches* or *localized pain* which might indicate a complication in sinuses, tonsils, ears;

Fever which exceeds the mild increase we have to expect in the beginning of a cold: 98.6 is the border line between normal and increased temperature which we usually do not reach in healthy days. Any oral temperature above 99.4 is real fever, indicating a complicating secondary infection;

Cough which follows the downward development of the infection into the deeper respiratory tract.

We shall devote a special chapter to these complications.

But before doing so we should like to take you first on a conducted tour through the office of the doctor you are going to see. We shall try to explain to you the instruments he uses, the methods of examination he employs, and the route by which he arrives at a diagnosis of your troubles.

IX. *What the Doctor Can See*

Nobody, except a hypochondriac, likes to go to the doctor. The reasons for the visit—unless it is for a check-up—are already unpleasant: something is wrong in the body, one of the organs does not function properly, there is pain; our health, which we like to take for granted, seems to be threatened.

The patient in the doctor's office who waits his turn—too often unnecessarily long—is worried. He fears a diagnosis that may confirm his apprehensions; he considers with misgivings the prospect of a prolonged treatment, and he dislikes the necessity of having to spend his good money on doctors and medicine.

In this uncomfortable situation the patient needs and should receive encouragement and reassurance. Most of it has to come from the personality of the doctor. A few words of sympathy can go a long way in creating the confidence that one's body is in good hands.

Still, faith in the doctor's ability and understanding does not remove all apprehension from the patient. Most of them do not cherish the idea of having to submit their body to the impersonal probing of a medical examination, to instruments, tests and other methods quite outside of their ordinary experience.

In this respect, the examination of the ear, nose, throat and larynx confronts the patient with a lot of mysterious instrumentary. Each step is done with artificial lighting and strange instruments, all in regions of the body which are hidden from sight and unknown to the average person.

A better understanding of the *technique of examination* is the best help in this situation. The patient who knows what to expect will feel much more at ease and will submit with better relaxation to an examination which requires good cooperation by the patient.

For this reason we should like to pretend that you, the reader, have learned the secret of the famous "invisible man." Quietly and unseen, you sit in the corner of the examination room of a laryngologist to observe the doctor at work. We shall remain at your side—authors are invisible anyhow—to explain to you what you see.

The room you find yourself in has the usual aseptic and utilitarian look of all such places. What distinguishes it from, for instance, the practitioner's examination room is the lack of the usual bright lights. The special problem in the examination of ear, nose or throat is that deep recesses of the body have to be made visible by artificial illumination. A semidark room provides a better contrast to the lighting effect of a spotlight, furnished by the head mirror. To increase this effect the walls may be painted in the pale blues or greens that are used in operating rooms too.

Near one wall stands a chair with head and arm rests for the patient and a small stool for the doctor. On one side of the patient's chair you find a lamp with a strong concentrated light. A table or cabinet exhibits the instruments for routine examination, bottles with different drugs, sprays, containers for cotton and gauze. An electric pump provides air pressure for sprays and other gadgets and suction for a number of uses.

Now the doctor enters the room wearing the *head mirror.*

Next to the syringe and the stethoscope, the head mirror is probably the best known of all medical instruments. But its function is poorly understood, at least by most cartoonists who draw it frequently, to the dismay of the laryngologist, in a wrong position.

The invention of the head mirror solved the problem that confronted Manuel Garcia and the early medical investigators of the larynx: how to obtain sufficient and shadow-free light for their observations. Garcia, as you might remember from Chapter I, made his first observation of the vocal cords in sunlight. Dr. J. Czermak who experimented in Budapest with the new laryngeal mirror hit on the happy idea of using a concave (inward curved) mirror to concentrate light from a candle. In 1858 he constructed the first *head mirror*. Since then, it has been changed only in small constructional details.

Fixed to a headband by an adjustable clamp the head mirror concentrates the light from a bulb into a powerful beam. The hole in the middle of the mirror permits the doctor to look along the axis of this beam. If you watch our doctor at work you will see that before each examination he swings the mirror into position so that the hole is in front of one of his eyes. The light from the lamp at the side of the patient is caught in the mirror and reflected—as a small but very bright beam—to the face of the patient. During examination or treatment the doctor has to hold his head absolutely still for steady illumination.

Now a patient is shown into the examination room. We are lucky because he is a young singer who comes for a general check-up. His teacher had the good sense to tell him that a professional of the singing or speaking voice should pick his throat specialist in healthy days and ask him for a thorough check-up of all vocal organs.

The doctor who has studied the body of his patient under normal conditions and has observed, on various occasions, his reaction to infections, drugs, treatments, is in a much better position to help than the once-consulted physician. The modern habit of changing doctors constantly, at the slightest displeasure or on the vaguest recommendation, does great disservice to the patient.

True, there are valid reasons why a patient wants and should change his doctor. But the "floating" patient who never gives his many doctors a chance beyond a few treatments is, as a rule, as badly off as the vocal student who runs from one teacher to another one.

In the meantime, the doctor has finished the preliminary questioning of the patient and begins with the examination. First, the *ears* are looked into. A small funnel-shaped instrument, called ear speculum, is inserted into the ear canal while the auricle is pulled backward and upward. Thus the **S**-shaped ear canal is straightened out, and the ear drum becomes visible in the depth through the speculum.

Next comes the *nose*. With your knowledge of nasal anatomy you realize the difficulty of examining the narrow cavities through the small openings of the nostrils. The doctor grasps the nasal speculum, an instrument with small blunt blades which are inserted into the nostrils and spread. The speculum keeps the hairs in the nostrils out of the way and widens the nostrils. To judge from the peaceful look in the patient's face it does not hurt at all.

Now, the doctor takes a spray bottle from the table, connects it with the pressure hose of the motor pump and directs a fine spray into the nostrils. Then he waits for a few minutes. If you think of our discussion of vasoconstrictors in the last chapter you can guess the purpose of the procedure. Under the influence of the spray the mucous membranes shrink and permit a better inspection of all the structures in the nose: the septum, the turbinates, the meati. The middle meatus (see Chapter II) gets special attention because there most of the openings of the sinuses are found. Freedom of air passage—

a necessity for proper function of the nose—is tested and deviations of the septum from the ideal straight line noted.

Few persons, by the way, have a completely straight septum. Even marked *septum deviations* are not harmful in themselves. They are significant and require correction only if they hinder nasal ventilation or block proper drainage of the sinuses. The conservative approach that has replaced the surgical enthusiasm of earlier years has limited septum operations to a few strict indications.

The rest of the examination of our patient is done through the open *mouth*. Our patient—a new hand in such a situation—hastens to assure the doctor that no instrument would be necessary for an inspection of his throat. The doctor smiles to himself because he heard this remark many times before. Quite a few patients have an intense dislike of any instrumental manipulation in their throat, particularly the use of a tongue depressor.

The reasons for this apprehension usually go back to childhood. It may be simply the memory of clumsy handling of a tongue depressor that was pushed with force into the throat of a struggling youngster. But sometimes the fear of oral examination emerges from deeper layers of our personality. As we know now, oral satisfaction or displeasure is an important factor in the emotional life of earliest childhood, and the adult resistance to oral examination is just one of the telltales that betray earlier conflicts.

Our doctor does not try to force his examination on the patient. We hear him explain that a satisfactory examination of the mouth and throat cannot be done without the help of some instruments, and that co-operation of the patient makes the examination easy for both doctor and patient. Finally he points out that a future singer—or any professional of the voice—will see his throat doctor more frequently than the average person. The sooner he learns to relax his tongue and throat in spite of instrumental handling the faster he will lose all apprehension in this situation.

Reassured, our patient submits to fate. He opens his mouth while the doctor presses his tongue gently down, out of the field of vision. The soft palate with the uvula, the tonsils—amazingly enough a number of patients are lucky enough to have them still—the throat, are inspected.

The *nasopharynx*—you remember, the space behind the soft palate—cannot be seen by direct observation. The doctor takes a small circular mirror, attached to a long handle, warms it over a flame and then holds it (without touching the throat) behind the soft palate. By turning it slowly he can now inspect in the mirror all the corners of the nasopharynx: the region on top where adenoid rests may be found, the openings of the Eustachian tubes. At the same time, he can look into the nasal cavities from the rear, thus getting a view of the posterior structures which are difficult to see through the nostrils. For this reason, this examination is called *posterior rhinoscopy*.

Now, the moment has come for that part of the examination which, to the professional speaker or singer, culminates the check-up: the *laryngoscopy* or inspection of the larynx.

To see the vocal cords and the interior of the larynx the *laryngeal mirror*—Garcia's gift to medicine—is employed. Larger than the postrhinoscopy mirror, it is attached to the handle at an angle of about 45 degrees. Before introducing it the doctor asks our patient to stick out his tongue and grasps it with a small piece of gauze.

The gentle pull at the tongue has a twofold purpose: it draws the tongue forward, thereby widening the space between tongue and throat, and, at the same time, it helps to elevate the epiglottis which normally overhangs the entrance into the larynx.

After a few examinations the patient learns to do the tongue-pulling himself, thus freeing one hand of the doctor for any treatment he might want to give.

Since this is our patient's first examination of the larynx, the doctor holds the patient's tongue with one hand. With the other hand, he guides the warmed mirror, grasping the handle like a pen, slowly into the mouth until it leans against the soft palate.

Our patient co-operates well. To his pleasant surprise he does not feel anything because the doctor avoids carefully any touching of the throat which is much more sensitive than the palate.

From your corner you cannot see much. Even looking over the doctor's shoulder would not help you. You would be able to see the laryngeal mirror in place but you would look at the mirror at an oblique angle and would miss the straight view the doctor has through the hole of the head mirror. In laryngeal examination only one person can see the vocal cords which makes the demonstration of laryngeal patients to a group of students difficult.

Since you cannot see for yourself we better come to your assistance with an illustration (Fig. 9). The light, thrown into the mouth by the head mirror, hits the laryngeal mirror. From there it is reflected downward and illuminates the interior of the larynx. At the same time, the image of the larynx is caught in the circular mirror and reflected back into the eye of the doctor behind the opening in the head mirror. The doctor *sees* the larynx.

Fig. 10 shows you laryngeal images as seen in the mirror. It is a kind of bird's-eye view from above. The epiglottis appears as a sickle-shaped roll (the upper rim), the arytenoid cartilages stick out as small buttons and the vocal cords are visible as white (or pinkish white) bands in marked contrast to the red of the mucous membranes which cover the false cords and the rest of the interior of the larynx.

While the patient breathes quietly the glottis remains open with the triangular spread of the vocal cords. Through the

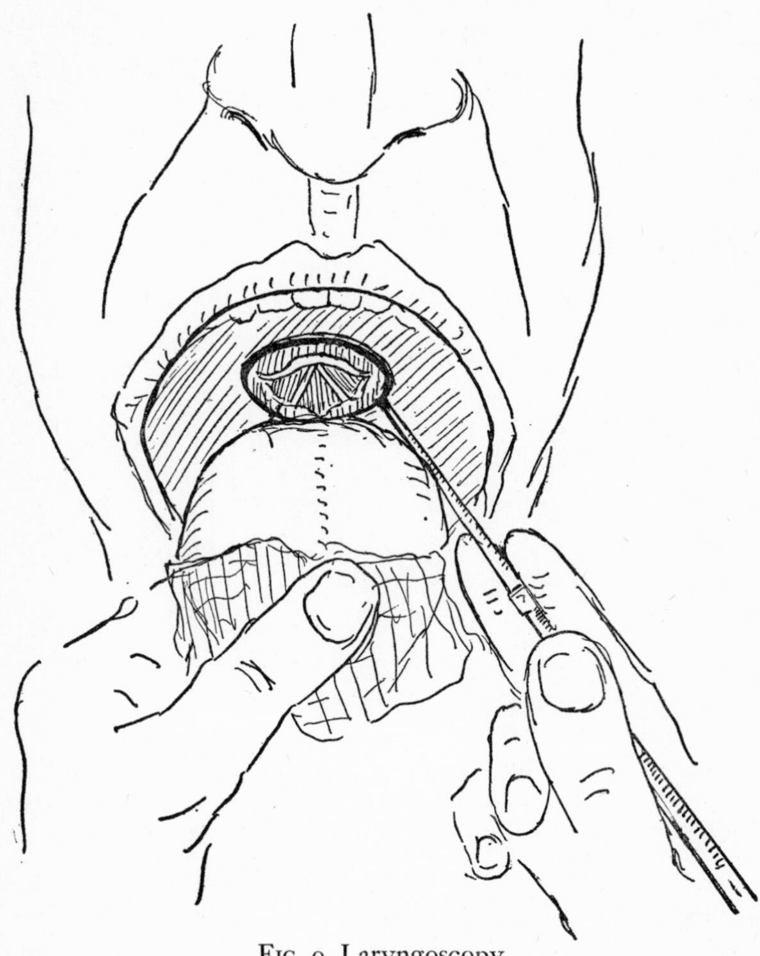

FIG. 9. Laryngoscopy

The left hand of the doctor pulls the tongue of the patient out while his right hand introduces the laryngeal mirror in which the image of the larynx appears.

glottis the upper part of the trachea with a few cartilaginous rings can be seen clearly.

To study motility and closure of the cords the doctor asks our patient to say "ee" with a high voice. This elevates the epiglottis even more and brings the cords into the position of closure.

As ingenious as this simple examination is it has a number of limitations. Since it presents a view from above, the upper

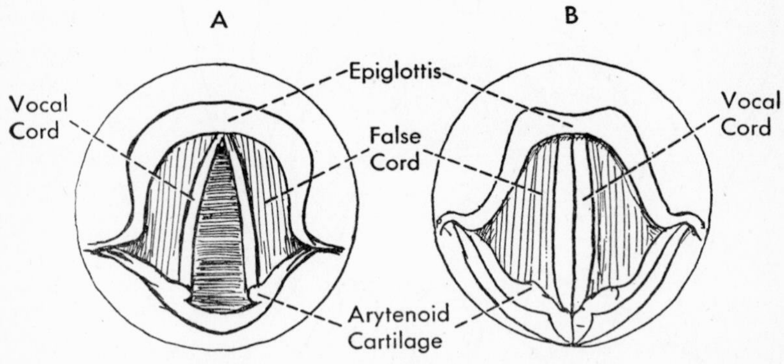

FIG. 10. Mirror Views of the Larynx

The drawings show the larynx as seen in the laryngeal mirror, A in the position of breathing with spread vocal cords, B in the position of phonation with approximated vocal cords. The circles represent the outline of the mirror. Structures seen above are anterior in the larynx; those seen below are posterior.

surfaces of all laryngeal structures are visible while other details are difficult to see or remain entirely hidden. For instance, of the vertical epiglottis only the upper rim is visible while the body of the cartilage can be observed only in glimpses. Of the vocal cords, only the flat upper surfaces with the inner edges are exposed while the lower surfaces remain always hidden like the other side of the moon.

This is a serious handicap because a growth that starts at

the lower surface of a cord can remain invisible and inaccessible until it envelops the rest of the cord or begins to protrude into the glottis.

Another difficulty is based on the fact that one does not observe the larynx directly but looks at a mirror image. A mirror reverses sides. As you see in Fig. 10, the anteriorly located epiglottis appears in the mirror on top, while the posterior part of the larynx with the wide spread of the glottis is seen at the bottom. Right and left are similarly reversed.

Finally, laryngoscopy—as all examination in ear, nose and throat—is done with one eye alone. We need the stereoscopic vision of both eyes to judge depth and distances. Looking at the flat mirror image with one eye, the doctor would lose all depth perception if he would not be helped by an intimate knowledge of the anatomical structures.

It requires great dexterity and constant practice to overcome all these obstacles in laryngeal examination and treatment. Using the image that appears in the mirror as his sole guide the doctor has to learn to translate automatically the mirror observation into the correct anatomical relations.

You can demonstrate to yourself the difficulties of *indirect laryngoscopy*, as the mirror examination of the larynx is called, by a simple experiment. Put your watch on the table, behind a heavy book or a small box that hides the watch from your direct observation. Then take a pocket mirror in your left hand and hold it, at an angle, over the table until you can see the face of the watch in it. Now close one eye, grasp a pencil with your right hand and try to touch some of the numerals while being guided only by what you can see in the mirror.

Most likely you will have a difficult time. Everything is topsy-turvy. The 12 is at the bottom of the image, the 6 on top and the numerals are reversed. Even telling what time it is will not be easy. And the point of the pencil will, in the beginning at least, refuse to obey your simplest directions.

If you now realize that the doctor holds the laryngeal mirror on a long handle, that he has to direct light from the head mirror to the laryngeal mirror and that all instruments used for treatments have to be sharply curved to follow the around-the-corner way of approach you will understand why even the simple laryngeal examination you just witnessed is quite a feat.

There is one way of overcoming some of the limitations of indirect laryngoscopy. By overextension of the head and a strong pressure on the tongue it is possible to bring the mouth, the tongue and the larynx into one straight line. In *direct laryngoscopy* a special instrument is used with a kind of heavy tongue depressor on a strong handle. Grasping this instrument firmly by the handle, the doctor slides the tongue depressor with some degree of pressure over the tongue of the patient and guides it over the epiglottis until he has a direct view of the vocal cords. Light is furnished by a tiny bulb at the tip of the tongue depressor. Local anesthesia is necessary for this procedure. Instruments for treatment or operation can be straight, and the eye of the surgeon can control their action without the help of a mirror.

Direct laryngoscopy is usually done in a hospital. It is used in the examination of patients with hard-to-see vocal cords and for operations on the cords.

At this point we should like to propose that we leave the doctor's examination room. The check-up we watched together with you was a good demonstration of the methods used in examination of the vocal organs. We hope it was sufficient to convince you that such an examination should not be faced with any apprehension. It requires great practice and skill for the doctor, but on your side only confident relaxation. That should be not too difficult for you now.

We propose to devote the remainder of this chapter to the

methods of *investigation of vocal function* that are used in research. Our knowledge of the human voice is a result of such studies, most of them done in the last fifty years. Their findings fill a whole library. We shall mention just a few of the more important methods.

One of the earliest and most fruitful approaches is the *study of breathing movements* in singing and speaking. While x-rays are very helpful in clarifying the movements of the chest and the diaphragm, they do not reveal much detail about the air consumption. To study this, the *spirometer* has been used. The singer or speaker breathes into a mask, the air is conducted from there into a bag which is equipped with a gadget that measures the volume of collected air, while certain notes or phrases are sung or spoken. Instruments of this type are available which register the flow of outgoing air as a curve on ruled paper.

Another method, called *pneumography*, employs an indirect approach (Fig. 11). Around the chest and the abdomen of the person to be examined inflated rubber belts are placed. Any movement in breathing changes the air pressure in the belts which are connected by rubber hoses to pressure-sensitive capsules. These, in turn, move pointers which write curves on the surface of a slowly revolving drum. You might have seen a similar set-up in the instruments which write curves of barometric changes.

Pneumography can be used to study chest and abdominal breathing in speaking or singing of whole phrases. In a famous book which Dr. M. Nadoleczny published in 1923 he offered the results of many years of exhaustive research of all phases of artistic singing. He chose characteristic parts of arias for his investigations and produced curves which show the breathing movements of good and bad singers, lyric and dramatic voices with great clarity.

The method is also valuable in the study of all kinds of ab-

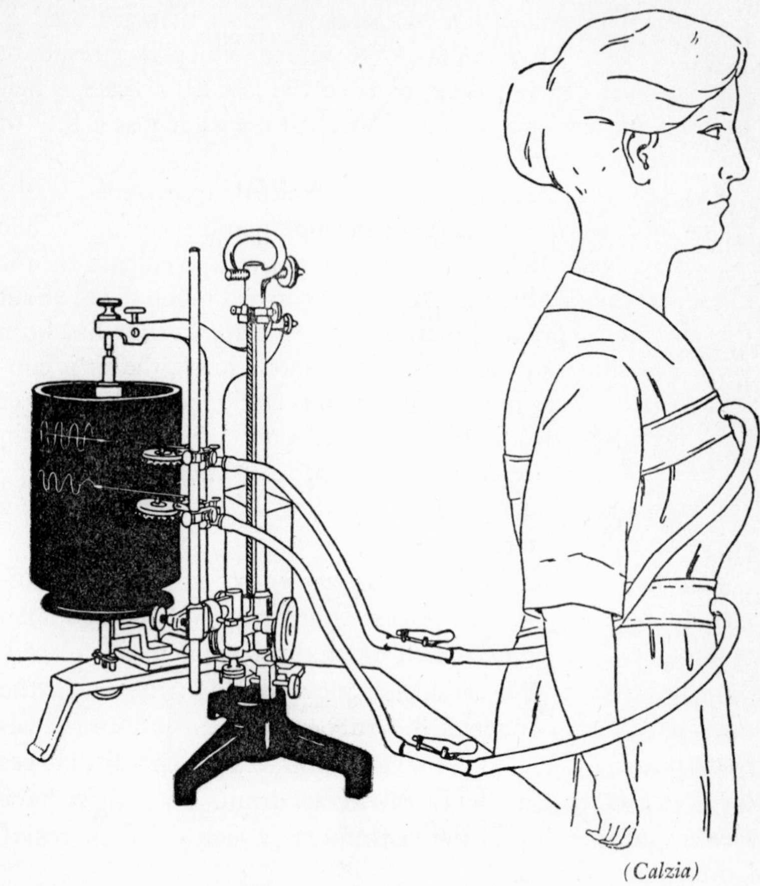

(*Calzia*)

Fig. 11. Pneumography

Recording of the breathing movements of chest and abdomen.

normalities of breathing in singing and speaking, and in disturbances of function of the vocal cords.

When you read our description of the vibrations of the vocal cords in Chapter III you might have asked yourself how any knowledge of these fast movements has been obtained. In speaking or singing the cords vibrate, depending on the pitch, at a rate of sixty to two thousand times per second. No human eye can follow individual movements that are faster than six times per second. This fact is used in cinematography where the showing of sixteen separate pictures per second are, for our eyes, blended into one continuous motion.

If we look at the vocal cords in singing with the laryngeal mirror we do not see any motion. The cords seem to stand still in the closed position. Their vibrations are too fast for our eye. To make them visible, an optic trick, called *stroboscopy*, can be employed. Between a strong light used for laryngoscopy and the head mirror that reflects the rays a fast rotating disk is placed with a number of slits which permit the quick passage of stabs of light. The disk rotates on the axis of a variable-speed motor. If the slits in the disk rotate at a speed which equals the number of vibrations of the cords, the cords seem to stand still. But if we vary the speed slightly we suddenly have the impression that the cords open and close in slow motion.

What actually happens is that each slit picks out a different phase of the fast motion of the cords. The eye of the examiner combines these single phases into one apparently slow motion.

Examination with these mechanical stroboscopes was very difficult. The patient had to hold one note at a very exact pitch, and the examiner had to adjust the slightly delayed or accelerated speed of the motor with the revolving disk very carefully.

Modern electronic technique has made possible the construction of stroboscopes where the voice controls directly the flashes of light. The voice is picked up by a microphone circuit which steers automatically a flickering source of light at any desired accelerated or delayed ratio. Only a few such instruments exist and are available for research.

In stroboscopy, the examiner has to keep in mind that he does not see the actual movement but the results of an optical trick which might be misleading in many details. Still, stroboscopy has taught us a great deal about a hitherto invisible motion.

With the advent of *cinematography* the goal of making vocal cord vibrations visible seemed to be within reach. But for a long time the technical difficulties could not be overcome. Aside from the handicaps that beset any cinematography of hidden regions of the body, no camera could be built which permitted the taking of pictures at the required rate.

Finally, in 1940, the Bell Telephone Laboratories solved the problem by constructing a camera which takes pictures at the fantastic rate of four thousand exposures per second. The experiments of Dr. D. W. Farnsworth produced a film of the human vocal cords in motion that is the fulfillment of a century-old dream. For the first time the vibrations of the cords could be actually seen, not in the trick-slowing of stroboscopy but as actual movement. The film which can be loaned from the Bell Telephone Laboratories for scientific purposes is a revelation to everybody who sees it.

X-rays have been used extensively in studying breathing movements of jaw, larynx, chest and diaphragm. To photograph the vocal cords by x-rays is very difficult because x-rays, during their passage through the body, register any resistance by heavier tissue they meet anywhere on that route. In the frontal position—which alone shows the profile of the cords clearly—the heavy bones of the spine blot out the weaker shadows produced by the cords.

Lately, a new technique of taking x-rays has been introduced. By this very ingenious method, called *tomography*, it is possible to bring a plane at any desired depth into sharp focus while omitting all structures in front or behind that plane. Tomographs are used extensively in x-rays of the lungs where they help in determining the exact place of an infection or a growth.

The same method has been employed to obtain sharply defined x-rays of the vocal cords without the disturbing bone shadows of the spine. Excellent tomographic studies of the vocal cords in singing and speaking have been made but the machinery is still too complicated for general use.

One of the best and most versatile tools in vocal research is the *analysis of sound*. In Chapter III we discussed the fact that pure sounds hardly exist in nature. All the sounds we hear are a mixture of a basic frequency, the fundamental, with a number of partials, the overtones. The German physicist H. von Helmholtz was the first one to study these sound mixtures systematically. With his resonators—sharply tuned to single frequencies—he could pick out all the components of a given sound. Examinations with this method were time-consuming and incomplete. But Helmholtz's book *Sensations of Tone* which he wrote in 1863 remained for a long time the bible of musical acoustics.

With the development of modern electronic equipment sound analysis advanced rapidly. The *cathode ray oscillograph* solved the problem of making sound visible. The sound is fed by way of a microphone into a box with a complicated circuit the main component of which is a cathode tube. The bottom of the tube is visible as a dark screen in a window of the box (like the screen of the television set). The sound is transformed in the cathode tube into an oscillating beam which becomes visible on the screen in the form of a luminous wave. This visible wave is not an image of an actual air wave but the electronically obtained record of a sound.

As such, these records are very valuable. They can be photographed from the screen and analyzed mathematically. The patterns of the oscillograph are as characteristic for any given sound—whether from an instrument or a voice—as the handwriting of an individual.

The newest tool in analysis of sounds is the recording of the *sound spectrum*. This is done by so-called *wave analyzers* which register automatically the number and the intensities of the overtones together with the fundamental. The readings for the fundamental and each partial are recorded on ruled paper in the form of vertical lines of varying height, according to the intensity of each of them.

To the experienced eye, these sound spectra or *sound profiles* show the characteristic sound qualities of each voice or instrument at a glance. The study of such graphic recordings has supplied the answer to many acoustical problems.

Voices of different type, open or covered singing and use of the registers can be studied and identified from their typical sound spectra. Dr. C. Culver, who has pioneered in this field, believes that the knowledge derived from these rapidly advancing investigations will deeply influence the methods of voice training.

We are still far away from a complete understanding of all the factors that go into the makings of a sound, instrumental or vocal. The teacher, the doctor, the voice therapist has still to rely on the sensitivity of the trained ear as his finest tool.

But there can be no doubt that we owe to modern acoustical research a wealth of new information that can no longer be overlooked by anybody who is interested in the mechanics of the human voice.

X. *Infections of Nose, Throat and Chest*

ALL VOCAL ORGANS ARE PART OF THE RESPIRATORY TRACT. Mouth and throat do additional duty as intakes for food. Nose and mouth are the only unprotected openings in the armor that shields our body against infection. The skin, as long as it is unbroken, covers all surfaces. The few openings are carefully sealed: the ear canals by the drum, the points of elimination by muscular closure. But through nose and mouth germs and viruses pass easily with the inhaled air. Infections of the respiratory organs rank high in statistics of diseases.

In the chapter on the common cold we discussed the mechanism of these infections. The virus of the common cold acts as the door-opener for germs of all kinds by weakening the resistance of the mucous membranes. The primary infection by the cold virus prepares the way for the secondary infection by bacterial invasion. Infections of the sinuses, the ears, the larynx, the bronchi are, in the majority of all cases, the second stage of the war of infection against the respiratory tract. The shock troops of the invading virus are followed by the regiments of germs which hold and extend the conquered positions.

But it happens, too, that a host of particularly virulent germs takes over directly without previous help of the cold virus. Streptococci, for instance, may overwhelm the defenses of the throat and produce a painful tonsillitis.

Infection of any part of the respiratory tract impairs, at varying degrees, vocal function. As a matter of fact, the disturbance of voice production is frequently out of proportion to the actual tissue alterations in respiratory infection. So complex and finely adjusted is the mechanism of the voice that any change in body sensations throws it out of gear.

For this reason a discussion of respiratory infections is in order in a book on vocal health. Of course, we shall not attempt any textbook completeness. We shall limit our description to conditions of special interest for the professional of the voice.

In discussing these infections we shall follow the same route as in our study of the anatomy. We shall begin with the nose and sinuses, consider mouth and throat and then—skipping the larynx—descend to the trachea and bronchi. The diseases of the larynx, as the most important one of the vocal organs, will require a chapter—the next one—of their own.

Since, in this chapter, we shall deal exclusively with *infections*, a few general considerations will be useful.

In medical language any infection from germs that do not cause a specific disease—such as diphtheria or whooping cough—are named by adding the ending "itis" to the affected organ. Thus we speak of sinusitis, tonsillitis, laryngitis, bronchitis.

Most respiratory infections are caused by germs of the family of cocci. Streptococci are the most frequent criminals, with staphylococci and pneumococci close seconds.

To the patient who cannot see the germs, the symptoms of the infection—such as fever, congestion, cough, pain—are the disease itself. Actually, these symptoms are the effects of the defense of the body against the infection. Raising the temperature—the fever—creates unfavorable conditions for the multiplication of germs in the blood. Dilation of blood vessels—causing the congestion and swelling of tissues—increases the blood volume in the infected tissues and brings a maximum of the healing forces of the blood into play. Pain—started by pressure of the swollen tissues on the nerve endings—makes the patient aware of the presence of an infection and forces him to rest the sick organ.

Even pus, the dreaded symptom of severer infections, is a product of active body defense. The white blood cells, the fighters of the blood, attack the germs in the tissues, dying in the battle by the millions. Their dead bodies, together with destroyed and still living germs and the remnants of tissue cells form pus, the scrap of antibacterial warfare.

The doctor fights the infection itself, while the patient wants to get rid of the symptoms. The doctor can accommodate the patient in his understandable desire only to the extent of making him fairly comfortable. He should not interfere with the defense mechanism of the body.

He can try to alleviate the pain by drugs but he should not depress the fever or reduce the congestion to the point where the self-help of the body would be endangered. Local pain may give important clues to judge progress or conquest of the infection. Forceful suppression of pain by powerful drugs may mask the symptoms of an expanding infection that requires surgical action. In short: the patient should always keep in mind that both body and doctor have primarily the task of fighting infection, not the discomfort it causes.

All the infections we shall now consider follow this general pattern. Their individual characteristics are determined by the special anatomical features of the affected organs.

If a plain nose cold does not end in the usual short course of a few days, secondary infection may extend into one or more of the sinuses. The symptoms of *acute sinusitis* are shaped by the unique anatomical situation. The sinuses are bony cavities lined with mucous membrane which are connected with the nose by small openings. The general swelling of all mucous membranes narrows or even closes the opening of the affected sinus and interferes with the drainage of the purulent discharge. The result will be increased pain, centering around the infected sinus (but sometimes "referred" to other parts of the head).

By pressing with the finger the regions of the cheek and above the eyes, the doctor gets his first indication whether one of the maxillary or frontal sinuses is infected. In maxillary sinusitis the close proximity of the root of the upper teeth to the floor of the sinus may produce "toothache" in the upper jaw which sends the patient mistakenly to the dentist.

Next to pain, the change of the nasal discharge from the glassy mucus of the cold to thick yellow pus is indicative of sinusitis. In examining the nose of the patient, the doctor watches for the telltales of pussy drainage from the sinuses. As you remember, the maxillary and frontal sinuses as well as most of the ethmoid cells drain into the middle meatus. Only the sphenoid sinus, which is least frequently affected in acute sinusitis, has its opening in the rear, near the posterior end of the middle turbinate. Pus from the other three sinuses will become visible in the middle meatus.

Of course, this symptom will help the doctor only if visible drainage exists. This is not always the case. The maxillary sinus, for instance, has its opening near the ceiling, like the overflow of a sink. Only if the whole sinus is filled with discharge, will pus be drained into the middle meatus. The frontal sinus has its opening at the floor, but it is narrow and easily closed by swelling of the membranes. The ethmoid cells are a labyrinth of small cavities, interconnected by small openings. Here, too, drainage is easily interfered with.

If neither localization of pain nor observation of sinus drainage gives conclusive proof for a diagnosis, transillumination or x-rays can unveil the place of infection.

If one puts a small electric bulb under the eyebrow or into the mouth, the frontal and maxillary sinuses light up in a pink glow, if they are healthy and filled with air. In infection of one of these sinuses the swelling of the mucous membranes and the retained discharge prevents the passage of light. Instead of showing translucent glow, the infected side remains dark on *transillumination*. It is a simple procedure which can be used in the darkened examination room. Its limitation is that it does not reveal anything about the condition of the ethmoid cells and the sphenoid sinuses.

For a complete check-up of the sinuses, *x-rays* are necessary. Infected sinuses appear in milky cloudiness on the film. Fluid levels of discharge in a sinus may be visible.

X-rays of the sinuses are helpful, too, in differentiating between actual involvement of the sinuses and *neuralgia*, as we call the painful irritation of the sensory nerves. Neuralgia of the supraorbital nerve (which emerges from the bone at the middle of the eyebrow) can produce pain, quite similar to that of frontal sinusitis. X-rays will decide the diagnosis.

As a rule, acute sinus infections are easily diagnosed. Infections of the maxillary sinus are leading in frequency, with ethmoid and frontal sinusitis next, and sphenoid sinusitis relatively rarer. All kinds of combined infections are possible.

What does sinusitis mean to the patient? There is definitely no cause for the widespread fear that sinus troubles are permanent. The vast majority of all cases of acute sinusitis is cured, with the help of modern drugs, without later recurrence.

On the other hand, acute sinusitis requires two things: medical help and a few days of complete rest. The latter is particularly important for the professional of speech and voice. He should always keep in mind that the whole respiratory tract is a unit. If one part is infected the rest of the tract is always involved, even if to a lesser degree. Infections spread easily from one area of mucous membrane to others. If we speak of sinusitis or laryngitis we mean by that term that the respiratory infection has centered around this or that part of the tract, but some degree of irritation is usually present in the rest of the respiratory system.

Complete rest creates the best conditions for fast healing of the infection at the storm center and gives the neighboring parts a chance to mobilize their resistance to approaching trouble.

In the case of sinusitis the danger of the spreading of infection to the larynx is particularly acute because of the constant downward drip of infected discharge from the sick sinus.

The *treatment of acute sinusitis* aims at: making the patient comfortable, establishing good drainage, fighting the infection and restoring normal function.

Anything that improves drainage and reduces tissue swelling will increase the comfort of the patient. Until that is effected one of the pain-killing drugs—from the milder aspirin to the more powerful codeine—may be necessary.

To restore drainage vasoconstrictors are used as drops, sprays or packings. Since the sinus openings are hidden in deep recesses, drops and sprays, applied by the patient, are not sufficient. In office treatment small pledgets of cotton, saturated with a vasoconstrictor, are placed near the sinus openings and left there for a while.

Frequently, this treatment which improves sinus drainage by shrinking the mucous membranes is combined with external heat by infrared lamps or similar equipment.

But the frontal attack on sinus infection is made by one of the modern drugs which have revolutionized medicine as few other treatments have done. The new age started in 1931 when the first *sulfa drug* (Prontosil) was introduced. *Penicillin* was discovered two years earlier by Sir Alexander Fleming, but it took almost ten years until this mold was tested in the fight against infection and produced on a large scale.

Since then, a whole family of drugs called *antibiotics* has been developed, all products of different molds. To mention the most important ones: penicillin, streptomycin, aureomycin, terramycin. New ones are constantly developed.

None of these antibiotics has yet been produced by chemical synthesis. They all are obtained by biological methods from living molds which make the production difficult and expensive.

The antibiotics—due to mass publicity and to stupendous successes in thousands of cases—are extremely popular with patients. They clamor for the drugs and—thanks to the weakness of human nature which rules doctors too—they get them on too frequent occasions.

Ours is a civilization of waste. We waste food as never before in history and we get vitamin deficiency in the midst of plenty. We waste big words which used to be the privilege of the poet and the rethor on the artificial excitements of advertising, and we lose our discrimination for real greatness of speech. We waste exaggerated emotions on soap operas, cheap songs and movies, and we lose responsiveness to the finer shadings of emotional expression. And we waste antibiotics—which, in other parts of the world, still demand their weight in gold to save the dying—on minor illnesses, and we get allergies and drug-fast germs.

To borrow and slightly modify a political slogan, the sins in the use of antibiotics are best described as: "too little and too often."

The frequent administration of these drugs for every minor infection is a risky procedure. It sets easily the mechanism in motion by which an allergy is developed. Such allergies are not only extremely unpleasant, but they eliminate the drug from future use in a real emergency.

Too small and too few doses are equally inadvisable. As every soldier knows one should leave a dangerous enemy alone or kill him. In administration of antibiotics, the fault of underdosage often lies with the patient. After one shot of penicillin he feels much better the next day and decides to avoid the expense of further treatments. The germs which were "hit over the head" by the first shot revive after a few days and produce a dangerous relapse. Worse yet, they have learned to live with the drug; they have become penicillin-fast.

The next patient who inherits the infection with such a penicillin-fast strain of germs is in a bad spot. He will show no improvement in spite of large and continuous doses of penicillin. The same behavior of germs has, of course, been observed with all other drugs of the antibiotic group.

Antibiotics should be handled as the big guns they are. They are useless in common colds because they do not influence the cold virus. They should be used only in severer infections but then in high doses and for a number of days. They should not be discontinued before *all* symptoms of the acute infection have completely disappeared. That is not for the patient to decide but for the doctor who knows what to look for.

If your doctor decides to give you *sulfa drugs* instead of the newer antibiotics, it does not mean that he is behind the times. The sulfa drugs which, for a while, had slipped into the role of the poor relatives of the antibiotics, have lately staged a comeback, due to their greater freedom from unpleasant side effects.

To return to the acute sinus infections: sulfa drugs and antibiotics are very effective in the treatment of these diseases. But they have to be combined with proper local treatment for quick and complete results.

In the medical era of "B.P.," before penicillin, the treatment of an acute sinus infection used to be a long-drawn and rather unpleasant affair, with irrigation of the sinus being the only active procedure and too many cases ending in chronic troubles.

Today, we do not touch the acutely infected sinus any more. We give large doses of antibiotics, take care of the drainage by sprays or painless packings, add external heat for further speed-up of healing and make the patient comfortable by pain-killing drugs. If the patient behaves and rests for the duration of such treatment, the vast majority of acute sinus infections is cured within a few days without leaving a trace.

The *chronic sinus infections* which used to trouble the life of so many patients are mostly the result of incomplete cures of acute infections. With the general application of antibiotic therapy they have sharply declined in number.

There is no need to go into detail in this book. A few facts stand out.

Chronic does *not* mean incurable. Even obstinate cases are now frequently brought under control. Where a complete cure is not feasible, at least the troublesome flare-ups can be successfully handled with modern therapy.

In many of these cases *allergy* forms the basis of the weakened resistance of the mucous membranes. Testing for allergy and treatment by elimination, allergen shots and antihistaminics (see Chapter VII) have become valuable tools in dealing with otherwise intractable chronic sinus infections.

Surgery of the sinuses—a frequent occurrence twenty years ago—is only rarely needed these days. The only operation that is still in more common use is the correction of a *deviated septum.* If the deviation interferes with the free drainage of a sinus, the removal of the obstacle by the relatively simple operation helps greatly to clear the chronic sinus infection and restore normal function.

Office procedures in the treatment of the chronically infected sinus include:

Removal of *polyps*, glassy bodies which are outgrowths of the irritated mucous membrane of the sinus. Removing them helps to re-establish nasal ventilation and sinus drainage.

Irrigation (washing out) of the sinus. While hardly done any more in acute cases it has its place in the treatment of chronic infections.

Before leaving nose and sinus troubles we should like to

say a word about that favorite of so many patients, the famous *postnasal drip*. Of all the complaints of nose and throat patients this is the one the doctor hears most frequently. Somehow, the public has been sold on the idea that mucus in the throat is a dangerous condition that should be fought.

Actually, as we have seen in Chapter II, all mucus produced by the membranes of the nose and sinuses is transported backward by ciliary action and finally wiped from the throat by the soft palate.

The pollution of the air we breathe in the cities, the irritation caused by the nasty habit of inhaling smoke and blowing it out through the nose and many other factors stimulate the production of mucus. The result is the "drip" of mucus into the throat. This in itself is quite harmless. So is the swallowing of mucus. The stomach does not mind mucus; it produces some by its own glands. And the acidity of the stomach kills the occasional germ caught by the mucus while it was still in the nose.

The situation is different if nose or sinuses are infected. Then the drip of purulent discharge spreads infection downward to the throat, the vocal cords, the deeper respiratory tract. If such infectious material appears in the nasopharynx or throat, the source has to be found. With the clearing of the local infection the postnasal drip of infected mucus will stop. But the drip of clear mucus should not worry you any more.

Tracing the infections downward we come now to the *throat*. There we have a whole group of organs which have a special affinity to infections: adenoids, tonsils and lingual tonsil. In Chapter II we described these accumulations of so-called lymphoid tissue, arranged as a ring, with the adenoids on top, the pharyngeal tonsils on both sides and the lingual tonsil at the bottom (see Fig. 2).

The function of these structures is still open to argument. They belong to the anatomical class of glands which are found in all parts of the body. Glands have the task of localizing infections and of preventing the spread of germs throughout the body.

The glands of the tonsillar group seem to be more important in earlier childhood when they help to build up general resistance to infection. The trouble with these structures is that their own ability to kill germs breaks down rather frequently. In that case they become centers or foci of infection which endanger health instead of protecting it.

The *adenoids*, because of their position in the nasopharynx, can cause a lot of local trouble. If large enough to block the rear exit of the nose they prevent nose breathing. In addition, the proximity of adenoids to the Eustachian tubes accounts for frequent middle-ear catarrhs and infections.

In adults, for whom this book is written, large adenoids are rarely found. But troubles resulting from infected adenoid rests are more common. If the removal of adenoids—usually together with tonsillectomy in childhood—was done incompletely, these remnants maintain a constant drip of infected discharge. The patients suffer from frequent attacks of laryngitis or even bronchitis. Careful inspection of the nasopharynx with the postrhinoscopy mirror will reveal the presence of adenoid rests, often embedded in scar tissue.

In these cases, revision of the nasopharynx under general anesthesia will produce dramatic results. After removal of all infected adenoid rests and scar pockets, the patient will suddenly be freed of the frequent infections of larynx and windpipe. This is, of course, a particularly pleasing result to the voice professional who has suffered, sometimes for years, from this hidden focus of infection.

Fifteen or twenty years ago the pharyngeal *tonsils* had—in adults at least—become almost as extinct as the dodo. Parents had been taught to ask for removal of the tonsils as soon as the poor children could stand the operation. But nature, in its stubbornness, refused to take the hint. Babies continued to be born with tonsils as standard equipment.

In the meantime, the enthusiasm for tonsillectomy has somewhat abated, both with doctors and parents. More and more children are permitted to reach adulthood with the tonsils still safely in place.

Most of these lucky people will go through life without ever experiencing any tonsillar trouble. During puberty an absorption of tonsillar tissue takes place anyhow. Healthy adult tonsils are, as a rule, small and hardly visible on both sides of the tongue between the pharyngeal pillars.

But occasionally, the tonsils are subject to repeated acute infections, lose their resistance and become chronically infected. In that case removal is in order.

If the patient is a singer or otherwise uses his voice professionally, the question arises whether tonsillectomy will damage the voice. Before answering this question we want to stress the point that *tonsillectomy* should not be done anyhow without the strictest *indication.*

Tonsillectomy is necessary:

If the patient has frequent attacks of *acute tonsillitis,* more than one in a year, or regularly year after year;

If the patient had one attack of *peritonsillar abscess* (so-called quinsy);

If disease in other parts of the body points to the tonsils as the *focus of infection.*

One attack of acute *tonsillitis* is not sufficient ground for operation. With sulfa drugs or antibiotics such an attack usually can be controlled in a few days. But frequent tonsillitis at short intervals indicates that the tonsils have lost their function as protectors of the throat. Then tonsillectomy is necessary.

Peritonsillar abscess—a common occurrence in the past—is now rarely seen. Throat infections are, as a rule, treated with antibiotics before an abscess develops. But occasionally it still happens that pus accumulates outside of the tonsil and has to be drained by incision. In that case tonsillectomy should be done later after an interval of six to eight weeks.

The third indication, action of the tonsils as the *focus of infection*, is more difficult to ascertain. Infected tonsils may look quite harmless. Size alone is not decisive. The larger part of the tonsil is buried anyhow in the surrounding tissues, and even small tonsils can be quite vicious.

The doctor has to pass his sentence on circumstantial evidence which often leaves room for honest doubt. Together with the family physician who knows more about the past history the specialist has to weigh all facts. If the patient has reason to believe in the integrity of the doctor he has to accept his decision in good faith.

Now, we can come back to the question: *is tonsillectomy dangerous to the voice*? Together with Dr. Robert H. Fowler who wrote an excellent book on tonsillectomy we believe that the answer can be given in the negative provided that a very precise technique of operation is employed.

Of course, no singer, actor or any other high-class voice professional should undergo tonsillectomy without absolute necessity. But if a clear-cut indication requires the removal of the tonsils, the patient should submit to the operation without fear for his voice.

He may have to go through a relatively short period of readjustment to get used to the changed sensations in his throat. He should plan accordingly and leave time for this process before he expects top performance of his voice.

Tonsillectomy is a relatively simple operation in the hands of the expert. It is not the easy procedure it is sometimes believed to be by the occasional surgeon.

As Dr. Fowler put it very precisely—in variation of the formula of the oath—the purpose of tonsillectomy is to remove "the tonsil, the whole tonsil, nothing but the tonsil."

The muscles which pull the soft palate downward run in the pillars which envelop the tonsils. In the tonsillectomy of the voice professional an extra careful dissection of the tonsil will prevent any damage to these muscles. If done with this precaution, tonsillectomy will not harm the voice.

The last member of the tonsil family is the *lingual tonsil.* We described it in Chapter II; you find it on illustration Fig. 2. In contrast to the adenoids and pharyngeal tonsils which often become infected in childhood the lingual tonsil rarely gives trouble before adulthood.

Enlargement of the lingual tonsil is probably the result of frequent small infections. It is frequently seen in patients who had tonsils and adenoids removed in childhood. The lingual tonsil grows later in life to compensate for the loss of the other tonsils, and then it becomes easily infected.

The patients complain about a foreign-body sensation deep in the throat, ranging from a "hair," a scratch, a lump, to—in acute flare-ups—a pinprick or pain on swallowing.

Examination reveals two large lumps of tonsillar tissue, deep down at the base of the tongue, touching each other in the mid-line. Sometimes, the mass is so large that it obstructs the view into the larynx.

Aside from being a source of chronic irritation, the enlarged lingual tonsil impairs the free resonance of the voice. The cushion of heavy tissue at the base of the tongue forms an obstacle which partly blocks and effectively damps the sound that emanates from the vocal cords. Persons who speak or sing with muffled or throaty voice should always be examined for enlargement of the lingual tonsil. It is a frequently overlooked condition.

The treatment of the enlarged lingual tonsil is surgical. The removal of the masses at the base of the tongue is a relatively simple procedure which can be done with little inconvenience for the patient. The operation not only eliminates the disturbing sensations in the throat, but effects frequently a remarkable improvement in the quality of the voice.

If a respiratory infection descends from the throat into the lower respiratory tract it may attack the larynx or become a tracheitis, bronchitis or, if it reaches the lungs, a pneumonia. Leaving laryngitis for the next chapter we can be brief about the rest. In a *lower respiratory* infection there is just one thing to do for the patient: go to bed and call the doctor.

A few general remarks might be in order. The descent of infection does not always proceed in that stage-wise manner. A day or two of a cold might be hardly felt by the patient when suddenly lower respiratory infection sets in with fever, severe cough and other local symptoms.

If a deep-sitting cough develops suddenly and temperatures go up it is high time to quit all experiments with self-treatment. The doctor should be called to determine the localization of the infection and to use what drugs he might consider necessary.

In a milder cough from the windpipe without fever, the patient may be tempted to try first his favorite *cough medicine.*

Cough mixtures consist of *expectorants*, drugs which enjoy a certain reputation for loosening the heavy mucus that accumulates in the air passages. To many of the standard mixtures, *codeine* or one of its derivates is added to calm down the irritating tickle that causes the cough.

Now, first of all, most of these expectorants—many of them great favorites with doctors and patients for centuries—do not stand up to critical investigation in the laboratory. Not one of them has any curative effect on the infection. At best, they stimulate production of mucus and help to liquefy dried discharge in trachea and bronchi.

Codeine is very effective in suppressing the cough reflex. But this is desirable only to a certain extent. To the patient, as we said in the beginning of this chapter, the symptoms are the disease. He is annoyed by the cough and he wants to get rid of it.

In this respect, singer and other professionals of the voice are particularly anxious to suppress any coughing. They are afraid that coughing may hurt their vocal cords. This is true only of the violent, hacking cough we see sometimes at the end of an acute respiratory infection. A mild effortless cough is part of the self-cleaning mechanism of the lower airways.

The cough reflex with its building up of pressure behind the closed cords and the subsequent sudden release of air helps to eject mucus from windpipe and bronchi. Keeping the air passages free promotes faster healing and reduces the danger of further downward spread of the infection.

Cough-stopping drugs should be taken only to the extent where a painful, harsh cough is reduced to occasional and effortless action. The vocal cords can stand a lot of such mild coughing without harm. Laryngitis is primarily an infection and not—as a rule—the result of nonviolent coughing.

In the treatment of full-fledged deep respiratory infections the antibiotics have their rightful place. Aside from administering these drugs by injection or in capsules, the *inhalation of nebulized antibiotics* is very effective. With special equipment solutions of these drugs can be converted into a very fine mist which is deeply inhaled. It reaches the finest bronchioles and penetrates even into the lungs.

The method has the advantage of concentrating high doses of the drugs on the infected membranes. But allergic reactions in mouth and throat are frequent enough to reserve inhalation of antibiotics for the severer types of respiratory infections.

The main thing to remember is that any extension of an acute infection below the larynx should be taken seriously. No lecture, no audition, no performance, no sermon is important enough to keep the patient from his more urgent duties of complete professional silence, rest in bed and medical care.

In this review of respiratory infections we have left out, as intended, the diseases of the larynx. We shall devote the entire next chapter to the troubles of the larynx, acute and chronic ones, to infections as well as to other organic disturbances.

XI. *The Sick Larynx*

ALMOST EVERYBODY KNOWS HOARSENESS FROM PERSONAL experience. To the average patient such an attack—if it is of short duration—is just a nuisance which does not keep him from his daily pursuits. But the professional of speech and voice fears hoarseness as a serious handicap and a danger to the quality of his instrument.

Hoarseness is one of those generalizing terms that resist concise definition. We looked up about twenty different definitions of hoarseness in textbooks and dictionaries and were shocked by the semantic carelessness and the medical incorrectness of most of them. In such a situation doctors like to hide behind a medical term. We speak of *dysphonia* which the medical dictionaries define as any impairment of the quality of the voice.

There is a reason for this confusion. The term hoarseness covers such a multitude of different conditions that it is without value for any exact description. Besides, we have learned in the last chapter to distinguish between symptom and disease. Hoarseness is an ill-defined symptom. It is the task of the doctor to find the cause of any impairment of the voice.

We shall describe only those conditions which are of practical importance to the professional of the voice. Even with this limitation we shall need a whole chapter for it.

The most common of all dysphonias is the hoarseness in *acute laryngitis*. By now, medical terms should not impress you any more. You know that laryngitis simply means an infection of the larynx.

In the vast majority of all cases, laryngitis is part of a general upper respiratory infection. Occasionally, infection attacks the vocal cords first. But, as a rule, some other parts of the respiratory tract are affected at the same time. If the nose or sinuses are involved, the drip of nasal discharge may spread infection downward to the cords. Or the constant cough in an irritation of the deeper respiratory tract weakens the resistance of the cords which are flooded with infected mucus.

The outstanding feature of acute laryngitis is the disturbance of vocal function which overshadows all other symptoms of the disease. If a patient has a chest cold it does not make much difference—from a purely medical point of view—whether or not the small area of the larynx is involved. As a matter of fact, the actual degree of infection in laryngitis is, in most cases at least, relatively slight. Pain, the symptom of severer infection, is usually absent.

If we look at the vocal cords of a patient with acute laryngitis we find there all kinds of changes, ranging from pink coloration to deep reddening, from slight congestion to severe swelling.

The latter is more important for the impairment of function than the change in color. The accumulation of body fluids in the cords which accounts for the swelling interferes with the free vibration of the vocal cords. Altogether, the visible changes in the vocal cords do not always correspond to the degree of hoarseness. It has been noted by many observers that very often a minor swelling and reddening of the cords produces severe disturbance of the voice.

As we have seen, the production of voice is a very complicated and finely adjusted body function which requires the teamwork of a number of organs. Any change, even a slight one, may completely upset this automatic co-ordination.

Almost twenty years ago, Dr. E. Froeschels examined the breathing of a large number of laryngitis patients with the pneumograph (see Chapter IX). The curves he obtained revealed remarkable irregularities of breathing. Both in speaking and singing, the breathing was uneconomical and erratic during the attack of laryngitis. After healing of the infection, the breathing returned at once to the regularity of normal respiration.

These observations are interesting because they confirm the opinion, held by many authorities, that the voice disturbance in acute laryngitis often goes far beyond the immediate effect of local inflammation. Somehow, the whole apparatus of voice production is upset during an acute laryngitis.

This general disturbance of vocal teamwork combines with the psychological impact of beginning hoarseness to create a situation where the voice becomes very vulnerable. As we shall see in the next chapter many permanent voice troubles have their origin at the danger point of laryngitis.

All this is of great practical importance. It gives added significance to the first and very urgent advice to the patient with an acute laryngitis: to keep *complete voice rest* for the duration of the infection.

Rest, as we have seen so often in these pages, is the outstanding prerequisite for fast healing of any local infection. To the professional, voice rest is essential to prevent permanent damage. His voice is not only threatened by the harm that any abuse may do to his inflamed cords. He must realize that he has temporarily lost the control over the delicate teamwork of his vocal organs. Any attempt to overcome this lack of coordination by force may set up wrong patterns of voice production which persist after the acute infection is gone.

The late Richard Tauber—one of the greatest technicians of the voice in our time—once told us that, early in life, he made it a rule for himself to cancel a performance, regardless of the consequences, if he felt the slightest irritation of his vocal cords. Observing this rule in his younger years—before world-wide fame made such decisions easier—was, he believed, a major factor in preserving the brilliance and technical perfection of his voice through a long career.

The need for voice rest is as important for the speaker as it is for the singer. As we shall see in later chapters, the damage to the speaking voice by enforced use during laryngitis may be less obvious but still lays the basis for many permanent disorders.

If we advise you to keep *complete* voice rest during laryngitis we mean just that. *Whispering*, as we explained in Chapter III and illustrated in Plate V, does *not* rest the voice. Persistent whispering of the "stage whisper" type may even strain the vocal cords more than conversational voice. If you cannot listen to your wife (or husband, to be sure) without talking back you better go into seclusion for the duration. Do not talk, do not whisper, avoid alcohol and smoking (the smoke from the cigarettes of others is as bad as your own smoking). With these precautions the laryngitis will be gone in a few days.

Since laryngitis is usually part of a general respiratory infection, the *treatment* we outlined in the last chapter will take care of the laryngitis too. There is little that local applications can achieve. A few drops of mentholated oil, directed to the cords by syringe or spray give temporary relief, but frequent use of menthol irritates the larynx. External heat—by heat lamp, short wave—or direct application of inhaled hot steam is useful as in all localized infections.

Laryngitis has the nasty habit of sometimes striking suddenly and—for the professional—at most inopportune moments. What are the chances of *emergency treatment* to enable the patient to speak or sing through a few hours before he retires to the necessary rest and cure?

One hears often about somebody's "miracle treatment" that

saved a performance. At the risk of debunking the glory of such achievements we have to tell you that in our field miracles are no more performed than anywhere else in medicine. First of all—as we shall see in later chapters—not every "laryngitis" is the real thing. Stage fright, first-night jitters, audition anxieties, election nerves and poor habits of speaking produce hoarseness that mirrors the symptoms of laryngitis. Many a sudden recovery at the appearance of a laryngologist in the dressing room goes under the heading of reassurance.

If the patient exhibits the beginning of a genuine laryngitis a few things can be done for him. Instillation of a vasoconstrictor on the vocal cords will reduce the congestion for a short time. A few drops of a weak solution of a local anesthetic may abolish the sensation of irritation and reverse temporarily the functional upset of voice production.

But no such treatment should be given without impressing very strongly on the patient: that this is not a treatment but an emergency measure; that vocal work under such momentary help may prolong the duration of the laryngitis afterward; that he should resist all temptation to force his way over still remaining voice difficulties; and that complete voice rest after vocal use under such conditions is twice as necessary.

Hoarseness in laryngitis should—under good care—disappear in a few days. If it persists, a laryngologist should be consulted under all circumstances to determine the cause of the voice impairment. If the vocal cords do not show any growth and move freely but exhibit the symptoms of chronic irritation we speak of *chronic laryngitis*. In this condition, the cords are congested, red, sometimes dry with surface crusts. On phonation, they often close poorly. The voice is raucous, harsh, frequently produced with considerable waste of air.

In chronic laryngitis the foremost task of the doctor is to find and, if possible, to remove the cause. Infections of sinuses, adenoid rests or the bronchi may provide a constant source of irritation. Excessive smoking and drinking, prolonged exposure to dust or chemical fumes, are other causes. Finally, the constant abuse of the voice may lead to a condition similar to chronic laryngitis. The barker at the county fair, the shouting auctioneer, the bellowing top sergeant, are typical examples of vocal cord damage by prolonged strain.

This occupational hoarseness furnishes an interesting example of the intimate connection between voice and personality. The professional who uses his voice for highly qualified and responsible tasks reacts to the slightest disorder of the vocal cords with a pronounced upset of functional and emotional balance. But the man who gets hoarse because of occupational shouting is hardly aware of it, even if his voice begins to sound like a calliope or a foghorn. His respiration is normal, his croaking may scare children, but he is not the least bit worried about his voice. He would not think of seeking medical advice, and goes through life, proudly exhibiting the roughness of his voice like a workingman's calluses.

So far, we have dealt only with congestion and swelling of the whole cords. If the cords are disfigured by a localized growth we speak of a tumor. In medical parlance any abnormal growth of tissue is called a tumor. The term covers a wide variety of growths, from the harmless corn to the vicious cancer.

A benign growth is well defined in its limits, does not invade the surrounding tissues and does not spread to other parts of the body. Such benign tumors do not endanger general health. The trouble they cause is purely local. They may cause pain as, for instance, corns do on our feet. Or they may impair the function of an organ by their presence.

This happens to be the case with the benign tumors of the vocal cords: nodes and polyps.

Nodes of the vocal cords are still a riddle in many respects. There is not even agreement on the nature of these growths. Some doctors do not believe that the nodes are true tumors but claim that they originate from obstructed mucous glands. Others have looked at them as products of chronic laryngitis. Still others have called nodes the corns of the vocal cords.

To you, these arguments are not very interesting. What *is* important to you is the fact that nodes of the vocal cords have, almost invariably, one single cause: *wrong use of the voice.*

Nodes are danger signals of the first order. They indicate that something is wrong with the patient's way of speaking or singing. Nodes appear because of abuse of the voice; once they have formed they create additional impairment of the voice by disturbing the mechanism of vocal cord closure and vibration.

The patient seeks medical advice because he encounters difficulties with his voice, usually for some time. If he is a singer, he—or his teacher—may have noticed uncertainties in the attack of soft notes. Or he experiences sudden breaks, usually in the middle register. The actor, speaker, teacher comes to the doctor because he is troubled by hoarseness after short periods of speaking. The voice sounds breathy, uncertain in pitch, sometimes with sudden wavering.

On laryngeal examination the doctor finds—at least in most cases—no or little reddening or congestion of the cords. But on the free inner border he sees the nodes, small, well-defined thickenings that jut out as pointed or rounded prominences from the otherwise straight line of the cords. Sometimes only one node has formed but in most cases they sit on exactly corresponding sites of both cords so that they touch each other on phonation.

They can form anywhere along the free border of the cords but, as a rule, they develop at a point where the middle and the anterior thirds of the cords meet. They vary in size from a pinhead to a split lentil.

On phonation the nodes prevent the cords from complete contact. The patient who is aware only of a difficulty in voicing is likely to use added force to overcome the obstacle. The result will be an irritation of the vocal cords quite similar to the one produced by laryngitis. Such laryngitislike changes of the cords are not the cause but the effect of the formation of nodes. And the nodes, as we said before, are the result of misuse of the voice.

Diagnosing nodes of the vocal cords creates quite a problem for the doctor. To begin with, he has to inform the patient of the condition of his cords. There are situations in medicine where a good case can be made for circumscribing a diagnosis in vague terms or even keeping the truth from the patient. Nodes definitely do not belong in this category. If the patient is a professional of the speaking or singing voice, the responsibility is too big for any softening of the truth.

Such a revelation comes to the patient as a severe shock, particularly if he is a singer or actor. He came to the doctor because he believed that he suffered from a prolonged laryngitis. Now he is being told that misuse of the voice is at the bottom of his troubles.

We face here a situation we shall meet many times in the next chapters. Nothing is so hard to accept for the voice professional as the fact than an impairment of his voice has a purely functional basis. He wants to hear—and may go from doctor to doctor to get the desired explanation—that he is the victim of an infection. Sometimes even the singing teacher resents a diagnosis which he considers a slur upon his teaching methods.

But the doctor has no choice in this matter because the only chance of undoing the damage lies with the correction of the real cause of the condition.

Fortunately, the patient can be told that such a chance exists if the treatment is planned correctly. If the nodes are relatively young they may again dissolve if the strain is taken from the vocal cords. In the beginning, the nodes are still soft, a circumscript swelling that can be reabsorbed. The older and larger they get, the more fibrous tissue is formed, making the nodes as permanent as corns.

Voice rest alone does not achieve any cure. Small nodes may disappear after a few weeks of silence, but they will reform immediately if speaking or singing is resumed with the same abusive methods that started the vicious circle.

Surgery as such is no answer either. It may be necessary to remove large nodes by punching instruments, but new nodes will appear as soon as singing or speaking brings the old strain back to the vocal cords.

The only effective way of dealing with nodes is to group the treatment around a radical correction of all mistakes in the use of the voice. All other measures have to be subordinated to the task of removing the strain that produced the nodes.

Temporary voice rest, particularly from professional voice work, may be necessary but reconditioning of the voice should be started as soon as possible.

Small nodes do not, as a rule, require surgery. There is a good chance that, with improved speaking or singing technique, the nodes will disappear. Large nodes of longer standing have to be removed. After a short period, needed for the healing of the cords, voice training has to be started.

A successful handling of the situation depends on good teamwork of:

The *patient* who submits to a complete overhauling of his speaking and singing technique;

The *throat specialist* who watches the progress by periodic examinations of the vocal cords;

The *voice therapist* who handles the retraining of the voice with methods we shall discuss in Chapter XIII. If the patient is a singer, the team will be assisted by the work of

The *singing teacher* who understands the implications of the condition and plans his instructions in close co-operation with doctor and therapist.

Polyps of the vocal cords are benign growths which may emerge from any part of the cords. They may sit on the cord with a broad base as reddish prominences or may be attached to the cord by a narrow "neck." They can reach the size of a cherry stone.

If a polyp originates from the underside of the cord or from the hard-to-see anterior end of the cord it may remain undetected, even on repeated examination. It may move up and down with the breath and become visible between the cords only on forceful expiration (for instance, in coughing). In such cases the marked hoarseness which a polyp produces will alternate with clear voice, depending on the momentary position of the polyp.

There hardly exists a laryngologist who has not had the sad experience of missing the diagnosis of a laryngeal polyp which did not "show up" and of being confronted later by the findings of a colleague who was lucky enough to examine the patient at the right moment. If he is philosophically inclined —as any good doctor should be—he will not be too depressed about his failure, and will not be too proud of himself if, the next time, *he* is the better diagnostician.

We still do not have a completely satisfying explanation for the emergence of laryngeal polyps. But it is safe to assume that chronic irritations (such as prolonged laryngitis, excessive smoking, constant abuse of the voice) are contributing factors.

The treatment of polyps is surgical. The removal of these growths can be done by the indirect method (with laryngeal mirror and curved instruments) if the polyp is plainly visible and accessible. In difficult positions or with an unco-operative patient, the operation is performed in direct laryngoscopy (see Chapter IX).

After the operation, every effort should be made to find and eliminate all possible causes of irritation. In this connection, special attention should be paid to the voice. To illustrate our point: the owner of a very noisy factory and a mediocre actress who both habitually strained their voice (the one by shouting in the workrooms, the other by speaking on and off stage with untrained force) had polyps removed. Within a year new polyps were formed on the vocal cords of both patients. Finally persuaded of the connection between vocal abuse and polyp formation, they both underwent systematic training of the speaking voice. No troubles have been experienced since, for six years in one case and eight years in the other one.

At this point, we have to say a word about *malignant tumors* of the larynx of which *cancer* is the most important one. We do not want to scare anybody nor to create hypochondriacs. But as long as we have no drug that cures cancer, everything depends on early detection. There is no excuse for the many cases of laryngeal cancer that still come to the doctor in a late stage. Nobody should be *hoarse for more than two weeks* without having his vocal cords examined by a competent specialist.

We doctors witness so much human tragedy which cannot be prevented or influenced that we hate to see lives being gambled away because of negligence or indifference.

Laryngeal cancer grows slowly and remains localized for quite some time. If the growth is still limited to a small area of a cord, the chances for cure by an operation or radiation are quite good. The remaining voice may be rough but is quite usable.

The trouble is that too many patients treat prolonged hoarseness with an amazing indifference. They would rush to the doctor if pain anywhere in the body lasted more than a day. But they take injury to their voice very casually. They seek medical advice so late that then nothing short of a complete removal of the larynx gives any chance of saving the life of the patient.

In that case, the patient can, at least, take some consolation from the fact that the loss of speech, entailed by the operation, is not permanent. A new voice which uses air from the esophagus can be developed by specialized training. Many of these patients learn to speak again with this voice which is amazingly clear and audible.

But let us say once more: cancer of the vocal cords can and should be detected early, at a stage where chances for cure are still good and natural voice can be preserved. There is no reason to fear cancer in every simple laryngitis. But a patient with prolonged hoarseness should be seen by a laryngologist at once.

To leave this rather gruesome subject, we should like to mention in passing two more possible causes of hoarseness: allergies and glandular imbalances.

We have discussed *allergy* in Chapter VII and mentioned it a few times since. We can be brief and say that any general allergy of the respiratory tract may produce laryngeal symptoms too. In addition, isolated allergic hoarseness occurs more frequently than it is generally assumed. If the examination of a patient with frequent spells of hoarseness exhibits a pale congestion of the vocal cords, one has to keep the possibility of an allergy in mind.

The same symptoms may be produced by a *disturbance of glandular balance*. Underfunction of the thyroid gland is an example of such a condition. Determination of the basal metabolic rate establishes the diagnosis, and administration of the deficient hormones will correct the imbalance.

So far, we have dealt exclusively with the possible causes of hoarseness. In conclusion of this chapter we have to add a word about *aphonia*, the complete loss of voice, by paralysis of one or two of the vocal cords.

The nerves which supply the cords with motion take a very unusual course. They are branches of the vagus nerve, a large nerve trunk which passes through the neck into the chest. Instead of going directly from the vagus to the larynx, they dip first from their origin in the neck deep downward into the chest, then turn around and return all the way up to the larynx. Because of this unique pathway thay are called the *recurrent nerves.*

This long course makes the recurrent nerves rather vulnerable. Any pressure they might encounter, by swollen glands in the chest, enlarged blood vessels, new growths, will damage the nerve and deprive the corresponding cord of its motility.

If a patient loses his voice and the examination reveals loss of movement in a cord, the search is on for localization of the damage to the recurrent nerve. It is difficult for the patient who consulted the laryngologist for his impaired voice to understand why he is sent for examination of his chest. He will be told that in this case the doctor has to act like an electrician who searches for a defect in the wiring to find the cause for the darkness in the lamp.

We have come to the conclusion of the second part of our book, devoted to the diseases of the vocal organs. Beginning with the next chapter we shall embark on the discussion of the functional disturbances of voice and speech. It is the least known, the most misunderstood and perhaps the most important subject for anybody who uses voice and speech in his work.

XII. *The Misused Voice*

MR. SMITH, A HIGH-SCHOOL TEACHER, IS A WORRIED MAN. FOR some time, he has experienced increasing difficulties with his voice.

We could call him by any other name because there are thousands like him: teachers, ministers, lawyers, politicians, salesmen, actors and singers. They all use their voices extensively in their chosen professions. Their work is specialized, responsible, requiring a high degree of natural talent, professional training, intelligence, authority. Voice is their great asset and, at the same time, their vulnerable spot.

Mr. Smith whom we present as a typical example is a good teacher who loves his work. He has an easy way with young people, his professional background is solid, his methods are modern. He is well liked by his colleagues and superiors. He is full of ambition and has good reason to assume that he is in line for the next free principalship. He knows that his superiors watch him for qualities of leadership and professional excellence. He tries hard to become a success.

But lately, he has begun to worry about the future. Slowly but irresistibly a threat has developed to his career. It all started rather innocently. After three or four hours of teaching his throat felt irritated, raw, scratchy. He had to clear his throat at frequent intervals. His voice became veiled, slightly hoarse.

He attributed his difficulties to a cold, stayed at home for a day or two, treating himself with the usual home remedies. He felt fine and in good voice when he returned to his class. But a few days later, his troubles started again.

During the next weeks, a nasty daily pattern developed. Mr. Smith woke up with a clear voice, confident that, at last, he had licked his "cold." Standing under the shower he even broke out into song. He went to school and, for an hour or two, his voice behaved well. But during the next classes all difficulties returned. His throat began to burn like fire, his voice became weak. The more he tried to overcome his vocal troubles by force, the worse he got. By the time he had reached the end of the day's schedule he was completely exhausted, hardly able to speak above a hoarse whisper.

It never entered his mind that something could be wrong with the use of his voice. He had always taken his voice for granted. At college, he had learned to watch his speech. He had been told to sharpen his S, but nobody paid much attention to his voice.

When he stood in front of his first class, eager to prove himself a good teacher, he tried his best to speak with a clear and loud voice, full of energy and authority. To go through a full day of teaching was harder work than he expected. Near the end of the day one became quite tired. But that could be overcome by putting more force behind one's voice. For eight years nothing had troubled him. And now, this prolonged cold had to hit him.

As a good teacher, Mr. Smith likes to rationalize the events of his life. In addition, he is a victim of the amiable weakness of his profession to fancy himself an amateur diagnostician. He has it all figured out: it is a cold and a laryngitis. What he needs is some good local treatment by a throat specialist.

He goes to the doctor, tells him the story of an unusually obstinate cold and laryngitis and asks for help.

The doctor who gives him a conventional examination has

no reason to quarrel with this diagnosis. He finds the throat reddened and dry, he looks at the patient's vocal cords and discovers the congestion and reddening of a mild laryngitis. He swabs the throat of Mr. Smith with silver nitrate, sprays his vocal cords with mentholated oil, prescribes an expectorant and recommends voice rest.

Mr. Smith feels better, goes home for a few days of rest, begins again to teach and—is back where he started. Nothing has changed, except that he has new worries: how to pay doctor bills for the prolonged treatment that seems to be in store for him.

If his doctor knows something about voice troubles he will change his diagnosis at the second or third visit. He will tell Mr. Smith that nothing is wrong with his vocal organs. He will explain that the real cause of all his troubles is a disturbance of the function of his voice and that only one treatment can help: training the voice.

If Mr. Smith is lucky he will believe his doctor and put himself into the hands of an experienced voice therapist. Chances are that he will fight this diagnosis. He will lose valuable weeks and months, going from doctor to doctor for heat treatments, short-wave applications, inhalations, penicillin shots, vitamin injections, getting worse all the time and slowly missing his chances of preventing the complete disintegration of his voice.

Mr. Smith might be an extreme case—although by no means a rare one. But functional voice troubles of all degrees are extremely common. To understand them we must now introduce the very important distinction between organic and functional diseases. In the second part of this book (Chapters VII-XI) we dealt mostly with organic disturbances: the changes of voice caused by infections, tissue changes in the vocal organs, new growths.

In *functional voice troubles* the primary cause of the disturbance is not a germ, a virus, a growth, but the *wrong use* of the otherwise healthy vocal organs.

In practice, the distinction between organic and functional disturbances is not always easy. Prolonged misuse of the voice may produce quite visible organic changes, such as the nodes of the vocal cords; or organic disease such as laryngitis may start the upset of function with effects that will become noticeable long after the initial infection has passed.

But the term functional disturbance is clear enough to describe a well-defined group of voice troubles and important enough to warrant a separate discussion.

Very little is known, outside of the small group of voice experts, about these disturbances. And almost nothing is done in the training of professionals to prevent slow damage to the voice by faulty use. The result is that few adults escape completely the ruinous change from the clear voice of the average child of two or three years to the rough, shrill, throaty or breathy voice of so many adults.

If we now try to discuss with you these functional voice disturbances we have to begin with the statement of two unfortunate limitations.

To describe auditory phenomena in printed words is extremely difficult. The most important instrument of the voice and speech therapist is his ear. It takes years to train it to perceive the often imperceptible changes that betray improper function of the voice. In scientific writing one can use accepted terms in the confidence that they are backed by the acoustic experience of the reader, gained through the observation of hundreds of cases.

You cannot have such experience and will have to accept some of our description at face value. You may be tempted—and we hope you will—to listen to the voices around you with an improving ear for the voice irregularities you will find in abundance. With greater experience you might even develop into quite a good judge of voices.

But you must be aware of another most undesirable limitation. If you try to judge the qualities of your own voice you are bound to fail. Even experts are often quite unaware of the shortcomings of their own voices.

We do not hear ourselves as others do. If you ever have heard a recording of your own voice you will not forget the shock of this experience. "Is that really my voice?" asks everybody who listens for the first time to the stranger who talks through the loudspeaker.

The reasons for this phenomenon are both acoustical and psychological. Our ears receive our own voice and speech sounds by different channels from the sounds of outside origin. And the conceptions and intentions of our brain are so strong that we may "hear" the sounds we want to produce instead of those which our vocal organs actually perform.

Having made these reservations, we can now proceed with the discussion of the types of functional voice disturbances. The voice can be damaged by using *wrong force*, *wrong pitch* and *wrong breathing*.

To consider these mechanisms separately means to simplify matters somewhat. As we have seen, voice is a complex process in which a number of different functions act as a unit. Disturbances of one part—at least in the majority of cases—affect the voice as a whole.

On the other hand, only the separate consideration of the single parts of the voice mechanism makes it possible to bring some order into the great variety of voice disturbances. All progress in medicine depends on the exact observation and classification of symptoms and signs of a disease. To leave this firm basis of scientific approach means to court the danger of getting lost in speculation and vague generalization.

The *use of wrong force* is the basis of most voice disturbances. In 1906, Dr. T. Flatau, one of the pioneers of the science of the voice, wrote a book, entitled *The Functional Weakness of the Voice*. With a great wealth of observations and diagnostic detail he described the functional voice troubles of the professional speaker and singer as a well-defined vocal disease which he called *phonasthenia* (Greek for weakness of the voice). Appearing at a time when throat doctors still thought only in terms of infections and organic changes, this book marked the beginning of a new approach to vocal problems. Since then, a whole library of papers and books has been written on the mechanics and the treatment of voice disturbances.

The term phonasthenia is still widely used. It is not a very good one because it describes only the last stage of functional disturbances which begin with wrong use of force and only end in weakness of the voice.

Dr. E. Froeschels has introduced a semantically more correct terminology by using the terms *hyperfunction* and *hypofunction. Hyper* and *hypo* are the Greek prefixes for "too much" and "too little." Hyperfunction of the voice means the use of too much muscular force—or of force at the wrong places—in the production of the voice. Hypofunction describes the weakness of the voice as the result of diminished power of the muscles of the vocal organs.

The value of this terminology lies in the fact that it explains the mechanism of most vocal disturbances in a simple way. Hyper- and hypofunction are—in a vast majority of these cases—different stages of the same disorder. It begins with hyperfunction, the use of too much force. If this hyperfunction continues for some length of time, the involved muscles cannot stand the constant strain any longer and hypofunction sets in with progressive weakness of the voice.

All the symptoms we described in the case of our Mr. Smith are only incidental to this basic mechanism. The dryness and irritation of the throat, the queer sensations in throat and larynx which finally developed to the point of real pain, radiating even to the breastbone, the roughness and hoarseness of the voice are but the consequences of constant speaking with hyperfunction.

No wonder that all local treatments did not help. They tried to relieve symptoms instead of attacking the disorder itself. If unchecked by vocal retraining, the voice of Mr. Smith—as the voice of thousands of similar cases—will slowly go from hyperfunction to hypofunction, ending in so-called *paretic hoarseness*, the loss of all muscular power. A weak voice, breathy because of incomplete closure of the vocal cords, will be the final result.

There exists a small group of voice disorders which begin with hypofunction. This is invariably a symptom of purely psychological origin. We shall come back to this type of voice impairment when we discuss the causes of voice disturbances.

Wrong force can be used at any part of the vocal tract. Dr. E. Froeschels has described six locations of such hyperfunctions.

The first one is the hyperfunction of the muscles which close the glottis. It is the *glottal stroke* (*coup de glotte*) which we mentioned already in Chapters V and VI. The effect of the glottal stroke is the hard attack of a note in singing, of a vowel at the beginning of a word in speaking.

The second region of hyperfunction lies immediately above the vocal cords. The use of too much force there leads to *self-strangulation* of the voice. The strong contraction of the pharyngeal muscles in the lower throat creates a bottleneck which gives the voice—both of the singer and the speaker—a characteristic constricted quality.

The third zone of disturbance lies a little higher, involving the muscles of the base of the tongue and the opposite part of the throat. Hyperfunction there is the cause of singing or speaking which sounds as if a hot potato got stuck in the throat. It gives the singing voice a rather unpleasant muffled quality which can be heard very often in singers with a poor technique. If you listen to the voices of your friends and acquaintances for these hyperfunctions you will be amazed how many of them speak with glottal stroke, self-strangulation or with the "hot potato."

The fourth location involves excessive tension of the soft palate, resulting in a flat voice without proper nasal resonance. The fifth and sixth hyperfunctions are characterized by stiffness of the tip of the tongue and of the lips. They are the result of overarticulation. Actors and singers who employ an affected manner of pronunciation are examples of this type of tenseness.

To make the catalogue complete, Dr. D. Weiss has added the stiffening of the muscles of the jaw as a seventh type of hyperfunction.

Hyperfunction rarely remains localized. It spreads, sooner or later, from the point of origin until all the muscle groups of the different zones are involved.

Almost all of us speak with some degree of hyperfunction, but, as a rule, this deviation from the normal, although esthetically unpleasant, constitutes no major threat to ordinary function. The fascination which the voice of a great actor holds for us is, not in the least, due to the fact that—without realizing it—we listen to one of the rare "normal" voices.

To the professional user of the speaking and singing voice any appreciable degree of hyperfunction is a potential threat because of the tendency to accumulate and spread.

The doctor, the voice therapist, the experienced singing teacher can make his diagnosis by ear alone. Hyperfunction, the transitory stage of mixed function and finally hypofunction in the various regions of the vocal tract produce quite characteristic voice qualities.

The doctor who tries to examine such a patient with tongue depressor and laryngeal mirror frequently gets his first inkling of the functional character of the voice disorder by the patient's behavior during the examination.

The well-trained singer and speaker are, as a rule, easy to

examine. Tongue and throat are relaxed and the cords visualized without difficulty. The patient with hyperfunction carries his habits of muscular constriction frequently into the examination. Without intending or knowing it he "fights" the examination. The tongue bulges, the throat contracts making the observation of the vocal cords possible only in glimpses.

The cords show—in the first stage at least—very little change. As a matter of fact the disproportion between the extent of voice impairment and the absence of any marked irritation of the cords is characteristic for most functional disorders.

Occasionally, a red stippling of the palate and sometimes the cords, indicating tiny hemorrhages, might betray the effects of frequent use of too much force in speaking and singing. Excessive hyperfunction may lead to more extensive damage to the cords. An actor, for instance, who plays a highly emotional part with uncontrolled shouting, may suddenly become quite hoarse. Laryngeal examination shows one cord with a deep-red surface, the sign of a *hemorrhage* from a ruptured small blood vessel.

In the last chapter we discussed already the *nodes* of the vocal cords. Their appearance is the result of prolonged strain on the vocal cords because of hyperfunction of the vocal organs.

In the late stages of hyperfunctional voice disorders when hypofunction takes over, the cords exhibit the growing weakness of the vocal muscles. On phonation, the cords close imperfectly, permitting the audible escape of unutilized air. This is the *waste of air* we discussed in Chapter VI.

So far, we have discussed only the mechanism of the wrong use of force in voice disorders and have neglected to discuss the *causes* of this condition. Functional voice disorders are still relatively unknown and have to be introduced first as an entity before one can deal with the "why."

The mechanism of hyperfunction can be started in many

ways. To begin with, we live in a tense century. Our civilization which stresses the spirit of competition as a guiding force transforms our lives into a constant battle for success. The general *tensing-up* which so many of us share can be traced in all parts of the body. It creates a kind of predisposition of all muscle groups for tenseness and tightening, including those of the vocal organs. The professional of the speaking or singing voice is an easy victim to vocal hypertension.

The almost complete absence of voice control and voice training in our schools is responsible for the damage to countless voices during the formative years. This neglect by our schools and high schools is, too often, continued through the training for the professions which require extensive use of the voice.

The young teacher, minister, lawyer, actor who has finished his training period and begins to work in his profession is suddenly burdened with a premature load of voice work which he is not equipped to handle. This *quantitative* strain on the voice leads to fatigue which the speaker tries to overcome with increased force.

Frequently, acute infections are the starting point of voice disorders. In the preceding chapter we have seen that in *acute laryngitis* the smooth co-operation of the vocal organs is upset, often out of proportion to the actual tissue changes. Trying to overcome this temporary handicap, the speaker or singer almost invariably uses force, and a new pattern of voice production is established that persists after the laryngitis is gone.

At this point, the deficiencies of poor vocal training combine with the effects of laryngitis to put the voice on the road to damage. The well-trained actor might be able to maneuver his voice around obstacles of acute impairment. But the professional without voice training is, at best, in good voice as long as no serious upset disturbs the automatic action of his vocal organs. The difficulties of acute laryngitis throw his voice completely out of gear, and the pattern of hyperfunction takes over.

Poor training plays, of course, a prominent part in the voice troubles *of the singer*. A good singing voice always achieves a maximum of tonal effect with a minimum of effort. Almost all the unpleasant traits of poor singing are connected with the wrong use of force. Lack of natural talent, the ambition of a lyric singer to invade the dramatic field, the lure of the high voices, are but a few of the many factors that establish the pattern of singing with excessive force.

But more than any other causes, the *emotional imbalances* of all types and degrees are responsible for the wrong use of force. The influence of momentary emotional upsets on the voice is a common experience. Under stress and excitement our vocal organs tense up, the voice becomes constricted, harsh, throaty, the pitch—as we shall see presently—goes up. Under the influence of prolonged nervous tensions, of neurotic conflicts, this pattern of constriction (the "shutting off" of the hostile outside world) settles on the vocal organs.

We do not need to repeat here what we said in Chapter V about the connection between voice and personality. With the professional of the speaking and singing voice, the vocal organs are the logical place for the transformation of emotional tension into disturbances of body functions.

There are countless situations that may cause and maintain this tight grip on the vocal organs. With Mr. Smith it was—among other factors—the ambition to climb the ladder to success and the fear to fail. The young minister who tries to represent authority in the face of inner immaturity and, maybe, struggles of his soul; the lawyer who pleads for a client of doubtful veracity; the politician whose existence depends on re-election; the actor in the rehearsals for his first important part; the singer who cannot adjust himself to the modest success of a choir singer; they all may become the victims of vocal tension. Emotional conflicts of private life—too numerous to discuss in detail—leave their mark on voices too.

An additional and important factor is the stress and anxiety *created* by the increasing impairment of the voice. A vicious circle forms: the original hyperfunction, whether from more mechanical or psychological causes, produces emotional stress which, in turn, leads to increased constriction and tightness.

In sudden fear, our voice becomes weak, colorless, low in pitch. Certain permanent anxieties lead to a *hypofunction* of the voice which in such cases, is not the exhausted end-stage of tightness of the vocal organs but the direct effect of fear and anxiety. It is another form of the attitude of shrinking away from the dangers of the world, of the inhibition of addressing the next man in confident sonority.

Aside from the wrong use of force, there are other factors in faulty voice production. *Wrong pitch* is one we have to consider. We mentioned already the changes of pitch under momentary emotional influences, the rise in excitement, anger or hatred, the lowering in fear and despair. Prolongation of such influences establishes the pattern of *wrong pitch* as effectively as the sequence of wrong force.

There is one time in life when a faulty pitch is established frequently. It is the adolescence with the change of voice or *mutation* which we discussed in Chapter VI.

In Fig. 12 we reproduce Dr. D. Weiss's scheme of *mutational voice disturbances.* The two heavy bars (4 and 6) stand for the normal development, with the male voice descending a full octave and the female one by one to two notes.

If the male voice does not descend but even settles on a higher level we speak of a *persistent falsetto voice* (2). The reasons for this abnormality are not always clear. Disturbances of the balance of muscular co-ordination have been blamed. But it seems that emotional conflicts are the most important single factor. The boy who does not want to assume the responsibilities of adult life, who prefers to remain "mother's little boy" or who inclines to female identification winds up with this high-pitched voice which may persist through life. In its extreme form, this is a very disturbing abnormality which makes the patient the constant butt of cheap

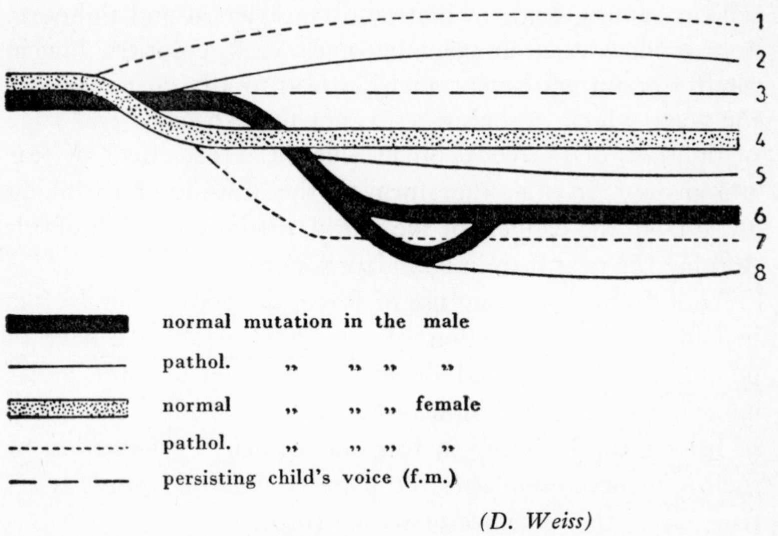

FIG. 12. Mutational Voice Disturbances

1. Mutational falsetto in the female. 2. Mutational falsetto in the male. 3. Persisting child's voice. 4. Normal voice change in the female. 5. Incomplete mutation in the male. 6. Normal mutation in the male. 7. Perverse mutation in the female. 8. Mutational basso in the male.

jokes. While the psychological situation which caused the disorder might be long forgotten and no longer valid, the voice disorder itself may create severe emotional tensions.

The most frequent one of all mutational disturbances is the *incomplete mutation* (5). The voice descends at the beginning of mutation but settles at too high a level. The result in the male voice is the pseudo-tenor which somehow lacks firmness and masculinity. The soft Irish tenor is a good example of it. Many people speak with this high voice of incomplete mutation. If they use this voice for professional purposes they experience frequently all the symptoms of functional disturbance which we discussed in the beginning of this chapter.

More rarely, the voice descends below the level that would be normal. This is the *mutational basso* (8), the artificially deep voice, assumed, for instance, by the future preacher who wants to impress on the listener a not yet existing authority.

The mutational disturbances of women are little known because they are less conspicuous. But they exist just the same. In 1899, Dr. T. Flatau presented a young woman who spoke with the deep voice of a man. Since then, this *perverse mutation* (7) as he called it has been observed and studied a number of times. In some cases, no reason could be found for the condition; in others, emotional factors seemed to be decisive. The first case we have seen was that of a young girl who spoke with a rough baritone. The identification with a cousin, a sergeant in the Air Force with whom she apparently had fallen in love, was the probable cause of the abnormal pitch. Voices are subject to fashions too. The imitation of the deep, husky voices of famous film stars and torch singers has played havoc with the voices of whole classes of high-school and college girls.

Lately, *mutational falsetto* with abnormally high pitch has been described in women too (1).

Aside from these mutational changes, other reasons exist for assuming a wrong pitch in speaking and singing.

In the singing voice, the uncontrolled singing during mutation or the premature beginning of professional voice training may lead to the fixation of the voice at too high a level.

All the emotional upsets we mentioned in connection with the wrong use of force affect the pitch too. As a rule, speaking at too high a level is much more frequent than the use of an artificially deep voice, for the simple reason that many more situations lead to increased tension and force with the resulting rise of pitch. Imitation of and identification with individuals and groups are important factors that influence the pitch of the speaking voice.

Finally, we should mention briefly the purely organic causes of glandular disturbances (3). Dysfunction or arrested development of the sex glands prevents the appearance of the secondary sex characteristics and keeps the voice at the child's level (just as the removal of the sex glands produced the voice of the castrate, as described in Chapter VI).

The third element of voice disorders is the use of *wrong* forms of *breathing*. We mentioned the functional upset of respiration already in our discussion of the acute laryngitis. All forms of hyper- and hypofunction involve the breathing mechanism too. In hyperfunction the breathing becomes enforced while trying to overcome the tension in the muscles of vocal cords, throat, tongue. In hypofunction the breathing may be shallow, with the audible waste-of-air escape between the incompletely closed cords. Of course, anything we said before about the influence of emotional stresses on the voice applies to respiration too.

Breath control is a special problem of the singer. Faulty breathing is very common with singers. Dr. J. Tarneaud who studied the breathing of a large number of singers at the Opéra and the Conservatoire in Paris claimed that he found only 25 per cent with really good breath control. Dr. D. Nadoleczny's pneumographic curves of the breathing of singers showed all kinds of imbalances of breathing, mostly on the side of too much force.

The trouble starts often in the days of the training of the voice. As we said before, there exists no set formula for ideal breathing which fits every singer. The singing teacher who tries to impose on all his pupils *one* form of breathing which his prize student found useful or which some famous singers are supposed to use will only risk the ruin of promising voices.

The best breath control in singing is achieved by smooth co-ordination of chest and abdominal breathing, and by a voice production which uses a minimum of air for a maximum of vocal effect. The preponderance of one of the breathing mechanisms is always dangerous. One of the most pernicious forms is the excessive use of chest breathing with raising of the shoulders and tightening of the neck muscles in deep inspiration. It is a danger symptom of the first order.

Faulty breathing, alone or in connection with vocal hyperfunction, is responsible for many cases of "off-key" singing. Control of pitch depends, to a large extent, on sensations of muscular tension. Any change of these body sensations disturbs easily the ability to find and maintain pitch at desired levels.

The same consideration holds true for the speaking voice. In public speaking, acting on the stage, faulty breathing with excessive pressure frequently starts the voice disorder which, sooner or later, involves the whole vocal apparatus.

Of course, organic changes may cause similar disturbances. Allergies and bronchial asthma tighten the small bronchioles, making breathing difficult and labored. Heart failure involves the lung tissues and impairs respiration.

A last word about the total loss of voice on a purely functional basis. In the last chapter we discussed *aphonia* from organic causes. In severely neurotic persons the conversion of neurotic tensions into physical symptoms may choose the vocal cords. The cords close well in coughing but remain open if voice is attempted. Such cases have been observed in great numbers during the two World Wars when soldiers developed this type of aphonia after severe shocks. It is seen frequently in very neurotic patients.

In contrast to the voice disorders which develop slowly on the basis of misuse of the voice, the functional aphonia strikes almost always suddenly. It is a symptom of what we used to call hysteria. The treatment of most cases is simple. All we have to do is to demonstrate to the patient—by various methods of sudden surprise—that he can speak with a normal, loud voice. That is usually possible at the first treatment.

With the other voice disorders it is not that easy. In this chapter, we have gone a long way from the simple "laryngitis" the patients like to blame for their troubles to the rather complex mechanism of functional voice disturbances.

All writers of popular medical books promise to give straightforward advice in simple nontechnical language. The trouble with nature is that it is almost never simple (otherwise this chapter would be shorter). The beauty and magnificence of nature lies rather in the co-ordination of very complicated processes, and voice is one of the most involved functions of our body.

By the same token, it is one of the most vulnerable ones. The treatment of voice disorders has to keep this complexity in mind. The next chapter will deal with the problems the voice therapist encounters.

XIII. *What Can Be Done about Your Voice*

In any medical treatment the relationship between patient and doctor is a major factor, deciding, quite often, success or failure.

In organic disease the situation is relatively simple, if the diagnosis is not in doubt and the treatment promising. The patient comes to the doctor with pain or other symptoms which plague him. He receives a convincing explanation of his troubles together with a plan for a therapy that moves along conventional lines. He might not understand all the details but, at least, he is on familiar ground.

In functional disorders of the speaking or singing voice no such simple pattern exists. Already the diagnosis—as we have seen in the preceding chapter—is made in terms which, to the patient, are perplexing and hard to understand. The treatment, as we shall see presently, is radically different from the drug-or-surgery type as used in organic disease.

Even more important, the simple patient-doctor relationship is, in functional voice disorders, replaced by the teamwork of a number of persons. They are: the patient, the doctor, the speech and voice therapist, the singing teacher. In some cases, the psychiatrist may have to be added. In view of the importance of a clear understanding of the tasks of the members of this team we should like to discuss first their work before taking up the methods of treatment.

First and foremost stands the *patient*. As a rule, he is deeply troubled by the announcement that no organic disease but faulty use of his voice is responsible for his troubles. He finds himself in a situation which requires a way of thinking quite different from the usual attitude of a patient with organic disease. He has to realize that no drug, no surgery, no local application will help him but that he has to go through a complete training of his voice.

The patient has to understand that this type of treatment requires time. Success depends, to a large extent, on the patience, persistency and energy of the patient. Voice training means to establish new patterns of voice production. It takes weeks and often months to form and secure such new habits.

As a rule, the diagnosis of a functional voice disorder is made by the *doctor*. Deficiencies of speech are frequently spotted by parents, school teachers, college instructors, but the troubles of the voice are usually discovered when the patient consults the throat specialist (as, for instance, our Mr. Smith did).

The throat specialist should be able to differentiate the functional voice disorders from those which have an organic basis. While this is relatively easy in very characteristic or more advanced disorders it requires a great deal of experience to diagnose functional disturbances in less obvious forms.

It is rather unfortunate that the medical profession lately has failed to take active interest in the treatment of voice and speech disorders. This relatively young specialty was built on a solid foundation of research and clinical experience gained by the co-operation of doctors and nonmedical scientists.

Dr. H. Gutzmann whose name is still remembered with reverence as the founder of modern speech and voice therapy was an M.D. His were a number of "firsts": first to write, in 1888, a doctor's thesis on stuttering; first to establish, in 1893, a regular course on speech disorders for the students of the University of Berlin; first to open, in 1907, a clinic for speech and voice disorders at the University Hospital.

Since the turn of the century, the study and the treatment of voice and speech disorders has been developed as a new and important branch of medicine. Most of the men who did the pioneering were doctors. The scientists who came from non-medical fields worked in close co-operation with hospitals and doctors.

To name just a few outstanding men: Liebmann, Flatau, Panconcelli-Calzia, Nadoleczny in Germany, Froeschels and Stern in Austria, Abbé Rousselot and Tarneaud in France, Bilancioni in Italy, Paget in England, Scripture in the United States. Everybody who learns and practices voice and speech therapy today stands on the shoulders of these men. He might not know it because the achievements of these pioneers are sometimes conveniently passed over.

Since doctors like technical terms the new specialty of treating speech and voice disorders acquired a Greek name, or rather two: *phoniatry* and *logopedics*. We mention them because you might come across these terms in books and articles. If you do not memorize them it is just as well. All these terms look impressive on diplomas, but otherwise plain English will do quite nicely.

In the last twenty years a new development has taken place, particularly in America. The study and treatment of voice and speech disorders has become separated from the medical profession. Every larger college has now a speech department where a steadily growing number of professionals are trained.

The great advantage of this development lies in the popularization of a new profession. Every year a considerable number of new therapists becomes available in speech centers and private practices to take care of the thousands of patients in need of treatment. The speech departments have become centers of new research.

On the other hand, the separation from medicine has deprived voice and speech therapy of some of the broader aspects which only a medical background can give. It has led to a certain neglect of voice problems in favor of the treatment of speech defects.

The blame lies mostly with the doctors. Only few physicians are still actively interested in voice and speech therapy. Of the 2,233 members (as of 1952) of the American Speech and Hearing Association only 19 are physicians. It would be most desirable if some of the younger doctors would join the ranks of their nonmedical colleagues in the study of the problems of the human voice.

If a throat specialist makes the diagnosis of a functional voice disturbance he has to decide whether he has enough experience to take over the treatment of the case. If not he will usually be able to recommend to his patient a good therapist.

If the patient has no such guidance he may have some difficulty in finding a therapist, particularly if he lives away from the larger cities. *Voice and speech therapists* (the official title is *speech correctionist* or *speech pathologist* but we prefer the term therapist which indicates partnership in the brotherhood of healers) are still scarce, and not all of those who work in the field have a solid professional background. *The American Speech and Hearing Association*, the national organization of the profession, has established high standards of training and practical experience for admission to membership and certification. The secretary of the Association (at present George A. Kopp, Ph.D., Wayne University, Detroit, Michigan) will answer inquiries as to regional facilities by sending from his files a list of accredited therapists and clinics.

While the doctor or the voice therapist appears on the scene only after voice troubles have begun, the *singing teacher* is already the adviser and tutor of the singer in healthy days.

To choose a good singing teacher is of utmost importance

to the young singer who embarks on an artistic career. Successful growth or ruin of the voice may result from this decision. Still, it is astonishing to see how often a singing teacher is chosen in a very casual way.

To judge the qualities of a singing teacher is, of course, a very difficult task. The student tends to be influenced in his choice by big names: either by the fame of a teacher as a singer, or by the brilliant success of a student who was trained by a certain teacher.

Both recommendations are, as such, poor yardsticks of the competence of a teacher. Some famous singers have become great teachers but not because of their artistic triumphs. Teaching an art is a task which requires abilities and experiences quite different from those needed in active performing. The great artist is often a poor teacher who forces on the student his own technique which might be excellent for one singer and disastrous for another one.

By the same token the choice of a teacher by relying on the big name of a famous student cannot be recommended. Some singers float from teacher to teacher. If they finally become famous the glory of their training is in great demand. One feels sometimes reminded of the seven Greek cities which, according to tradition, fought for the claim to be the birthplace of Homer.

The good singing teacher is, first and last, a teacher of born abilities which are rather rare. He has to have the true teacher's instinct, backed by thorough training and wide experience, of adapting his methods to the individual characteristics, physical and mental, of each new student. He has to be a first-class musician. And he has to know enough about the technique, the mechanics, the acoustics and the psychology of singing to build his teaching methods on a firm basis of modern science.

The success of a teacher with a large number of different students is probably the best recommendation. The average quality of many good students with all types of voices and personalities counts more than the lucky single star pupil.

The poor qualifications of too many teachers have worried the profession for a long time. The *National Association of Teachers of Singing* has striven hard to raise the standards of teaching. Its requirements for membership are high. As of 1952, 1,443 singing teachers have been admitted. The eight districts and a large number of local branches of the Association offer to their members opportunities for study through lectures and workshops which present the advances of science and teaching practice.

If local advice is unobtainable in the choice of a good singing teacher the secretary of the Association (5040 North St. Louis Street, Chicago, Illinois) will furnish the inquirer with a list of members in the city of his residence.

If a singer develops voice troubles the close co-operation between singing teacher and doctor or therapist is of utmost importance. The successful handling of functional voice disorders in singers depends on this teamwork which is frequently missing. Doctors often know too little about the special problems of singing, and the singing teachers resent frequently any interference into what they consider their proper domain.

Very often, the doctor finds himself in a difficult spot. He may suspect that poor teaching is a major factor in the development of a voice disturbance but hesitates, for obvious reasons, to say so. Handling such situations successfully without offending the patient and antagonizing the teacher is an excellent training for the diplomatic career.

The therapists are not much help either because they are so occupied with speech correction work that they do not pay enough attention to the disorders of the singing voice.

In well-co-ordinated teamwork the doctor should diagnose the functional character of a voice disturbance, and should then proceed to plan the proper treatment. The singing teacher should know that in many functional disorders treatment with special methods by doctor or therapist has to be given before regular voice training can be safely resumed. The more each member of the team knows about the field of the other, the better the chances of the patient for complete recovery.

In the preceding chapter we have seen that emotional problems and conflicts play an important part in the development of voice disorders. What help can *psychotherapy* give in the treatment of these conditions?

A simple answer can be given only in the relatively small group of cases where the voice disturbance is merely a symptom of a severe neurosis or a psychosis. These cases clearly belong in the hands of the psychiatrist.

The vast majority of voice disorders contains both mechanical and psychological elements in varying mixtures, from preponderantly technical misuse of the voice with rather superficial emotional implications to disturbances with a decidedly neurotic or even psychotic basis.

If the neurotic element is too strong to be neglected the help of a psychiatrist or analyst would be valuable. But psychotherapists are still limited in number and too overburdened with work to be easily available. In addition, the handling of voice cases requires specialized training. As a rule, psychotherapists lack the experience which is needed to judge and control disorders of voice and speech. They are, therefore, reluctant to accept such cases.

Finally, psychotherapy does not always provide the answer to the problems of the voice. Successful removal of emotional conflicts which started the pattern of voice disorders does not automatically correct the pattern of misuse which has become firmly established.

Personal preference and conviction of the voice therapist will decide whether the treatment of a given case should be planned around the correction of the misuse of the voice or be based on the attempt to evaluate and influence the psychological basis.

The majority of cases will respond quite satisfactorily to a more technical approach. As a rule, the professional of the singing or speaking voice is better off if his vocal function is made as independent as possible of his personal emotional experience. It is preferable—and usually feasible—to break into the vicious circle of psychologically caused voice disorder from the side of the voice.

In addition, voice therapy has very often a definite psychotherapeutic effect. It is fascinating to note the marked change in personality which develops frequently as a by-product of an improved use of the voice.

Of course, all that does not mean that any good therapist will neglect to study and note the psychological background of a given case. Where the various schools of therapists disagree is on the question of what use should be made of such insight into the emotional undertow of a voice disorder. Keeping such knowledge from the patient during a treatment does not mean to deny the importance of the emotional factor. In disturbances of a body function as personal as the voice any kind of treatment contains a strong psychotherapeutic element. In the last resort, it is the personality of the therapist which decides the success of treatment.

Is *self-treatment* of voice disorders possible? Only to a very limited extent. The most important step in any voice treatment is to come to a correct diagnosis. We have seen that, because of the inability of judging his own voice objectively, the patient needs outside expert help in being made aware of the troubles that beset him. The same holds true for the treatment.

All the well-meaning formulas we read so often in articles and books for acquiring a "pleasant" or "strong" voice fail to take notice of the dangers and grave risks that self-doctoring of the voice implies.

On the other hand, the goal of any sound voice treatment must be to let the patient stand on his own feet as soon as possible. A treatment that does not achieve this defeats its own purpose. But the reconditioning of the voice is a process that cannot be completed in a few easy lessons. The longer the misuse of the voice has been going on, the harder it will be to break the faulty patterns and to guide the voice back to normalized production.

If one would believe the teachings of many of the popular books on speaking and singing all that is needed is to learn how to "relax." Few words have lost so much of their meaning by constant and uncritical overuse as *relaxation.* If we had our way we would recommend to Congress the passing of a law forbidding the use of the word relaxation for a few years. In our supercharged civilization people try so hard to relax that they become tense all over.

Using our vocal organs for the production of voice and speech is an *active* function of the body. Any action of muscles is based on varying degrees of tension (or tonus as the physiologists call it). The secret of normal function is not relaxation (which is complete only in death) but the use of the *right* muscles and the application of the *right* degree of muscle tonus.

Since the majority of voice troubles results from exaggerated muscle activity, the first duty of the therapist is to see that this hyperfunction is reduced.

This can be achieved by attacking the local symptoms or by dealing with vocal function as a unit. A very useful procedure to overcome stiffness of the jaw, strangulating tightness of the throat and tongue is the so-called *shaking of the jaw* which has become an accepted exercise with many singing teachers. While the mouth is kept slightly open and a voice sound produced, the jaw is moved loosely and rapidly from side to side. If done correctly this exercise goes a long way in breaking up the grip of tightness on the voice.

Local manipulations, as recommended by some teachers, should be avoided. They create only new hyperfunctions which may be more dangerous than the troubles they are supposed to overcome.

An exception to this rule is the application of pressure on the thyroid cartilage which is sometimes used to suddenly lower the pitch of a high speaking voice. Pressing with the finger on the cartilage with a slight backward-downward push reduces the tension of the vocal cords and brings the voice level down. It is used only as an initial procedure which demonstrates to the patient his ability to speak with a lower voice. Once that purpose has been achieved the patient is taught to speak in a normal voice without such artificial help.

Various methods have been used to strengthen muscular action in marked *hypofunction* of the voice. A weak *faradic current* passed through the neck at the height of the vocal cords raises the pitch of a given sound. Complicated machines have been constructed to combine the effect of the electric current with the tuning-up stimulation of massage. Vibration massage has been synchronized with the vibrations of the vocal cords. While helpful in some cases it is hard to determine how much of the result achieved is due to the physical therapy or to the psychological impact of an impressive gadget.

In marked hypofunction or in loss of the voice (*aphonia*), due to damage to the recurrent nerve, the *pushing exercises*, as introduced by Froeschels, are very effective. They are based on the fact that sudden tensing of the muscles which move the arm downward stimulates the tonus of the vocal muscles too. The fists are brought down from the chest—at the height of the nipples—in a forceful manner while, at the same time, a vowel is voiced preceded by a consonant (for instance, P-Ah, P-A, P-O). Perfect synchronization between the push and the voicing is important.

The method is being used in the treatment of many forms of muscular weaknesses: to strengthen palatal action in hypernasality, normalize the voice in hypofunction, stimulate lost motion of vocal cords.

All commonly used methods which try to correct a faulty use of the voice by some kind of specialized exercise have a common disadvantage. They focus the attention of the patient on the part of the vocal tract around which the disturbance centers, make him overly conscious of the sensations and tensions in these regions.

This is the common mistake of such recommendations as: dropping the jaw, flattening the tongue, directing the tone to certain parts of the vocal tract. All these methods are based on the misconception that a "normal" pattern of positions or motions can be established that fits every voice. A treatment which would restore vocal health without paying conscious attention to single elements of voice production would be superior to all forms of such "exercise."

Such an approach was introduced by Dr. E. Froeschels who based his treatment of voice disorders and—as we shall see—of some speech defects on the use of chewing.

The function of *chewing* is a twin of speaking. We use the same muscles in chewing and speaking. Moreover—and that makes it a unique phenomenon—we can speak and chew at the same time.

Dr. Froeschels believes that human speech has, from the early days of mankind, developed out of chewing noises. Of course, no positive proof can be obtained for any explanation of a body function that emerged long before recorded history. But it seems that, thousands of years ago, the dim memory of a common origin of both functions was still alive. In the hieroglyphic script of the old Egyptians the same picture-sign was used both for speaking and eating: a kneeling man who points a finger to his mouth.

Even in pronounced disturbances of the voice the smoothness and ease of the chewing movements is preserved. In using the motion of chewing for voice production the therapist appeals to an inborn function which transfers the undisturbed muscular teamwork of chewing to the motions of voiced speech.

Chewing consists of more than the chopping up-and-down movements of the jaw. The tongue moves continuously in a completely irregular pattern. X-ray films of chewing have demonstrated that all the muscles, down to the larynx, are involved in an easy rhythm of flowing motion.

Since its introduction, nineteen years ago, the chewing method has been tested and found extremely useful by a number of therapists. Their experiences are reported in a book by Dr. D. Weiss and H. Beebe which should be consulted for greater detail (see list of recommended reading).

In a typical treatment the patient is first given a short explanation. He is reminded of the fact that we can chew and speak at the same time, and is told that primitive people still chew aloud with open lips.

The patient is then asked to concentrate on the idea that he is eating and to chew "like a savage," opening the mouth slightly and with extensive movements of the lips and the tongue. Finally, he is asked to give voice while the chewing continues.

If done correctly a great variety of sounds is formed. People who listen to a recording of such voiced chewing of another person almost invariably have the impression of being confronted with a strange language.

The most frequent mistakes patients make in the beginning is to slip into a stereotyped jaw motion with the tongue lying flat at the floor of the mouth. A monotonous "yam-yam-yam" results. Only during chewing with lively free movements of the tongue is the desirable variety of speech sounds produced. Sometimes the chewing of a piece of bread has to be used to make the patient aware of the tongue movements in actual eating, but this practice should be abandoned as soon as possible in favor of concentrating on the *idea* of chewing.

Since the formation of a new pattern requires constant repetition, the patient is instructed to practice chewing at least twenty times daily for a few seconds each time.

With greater perfection of voiced chewing being reached, speech is slowly added. At this stage the exaggerated chewing can be tuned down to the point where the speaker is still aware of chewing motions but an uninformed listener would not notice them any more.

The method has been used by a number of famous actors, singers, preachers and teachers with very good results.

The effect of the first correct chewing on the character of the voice is sometimes startling. The constricted voice of hyperfunction gives way to a free voice production of pleasant character. One has the impression that the normal voice has been restored by a natural process.

A similar effect can be observed on the pitch of speaking. Changing the too-high or too-low pitch of a patient is not difficult for the experienced therapist. The problem is only at what level the pitch should be considered as normal. To leave this decision to the subjective preference of the therapist is a risky procedure. Chewing is a valuable aid in establishing the natural level of a speaking voice. Under the effect of correct chewing the voice rises or descends until it has "found home."

The great advantage of the chewing method is that it activates an easily available and always undisturbed function. In using this twin function for the speaking voice one is able to bypass the emotional tensions which have burdened the voice. As G. L. Wyatt has pointed out, in chewing a tone the patient abandons temporarily the communicative character of speech and returns to vocal play, the earliest form of vocal activity.

For this reason, chewing should not be called an "exercise." Instead of focusing the attention of the patient on a single symptom, as all the conventional exercises do, he should become convinced that he uses a completely new approach to voice production.

That does not mean that the chewing technique is a simple tool for self-treatment. As any other voice therapy it requires supervision by an experienced therapist who controls the correct approach in the beginning and guides later the transition to "normal" speaking. In the treatment of disorders of the singing voice the chewing technique helps to establish a normalized basis for sound production upon which the singing teacher can then proceed to build a safe singing technique.

One element of voice production that requires special attention in voice disorders of professionals is the control of breathing. In the preceding chapter we mentioned the great frequency of faulty breathing in speakers and singers. The *correction of poor breathing habits* has a twofold goal: to teach the patient the use of utmost economy of breath and to establish chest and abdominal breathing as an integrated function.

Economy of breathing means economy of expiration. The training of breathing is a keystone of the education of a singer. Still, perfect and economical expiration is an exception with singers rather than the rule. With public speakers of all kinds matters are even worse. The cutting-up of sentences because of shallow or pressed breathing, and waste of air is so frequent that one hardly notices it any more.

Successful training by methods designed to correct hyper- or hypofunction goes a long way to improve breathing. Still, additional training of breathing is necessary in many cases.

One of the simplest exercises to improve economy of expiration consists of slow but steady expiration with open mouth on a voiceless H-sound. A well-trained person should be able to continue such expiration for, at least, thirty to forty-five seconds. To prevent stiffness and jerkiness, the exercise is best performed standing up with sideward raising of the arms to the horizonal at deep inspiration and slow lowering during expiration.

The breathing of many patients is so poor that it collapses

after ten or fifteen seconds. In that case it is advisable to start these exercises with expiration on an F or S sound which is easier because of the frictional resistance of these sounds. The exercise should not be performed more than three times in a row because, if done in excess, it might become a strain on the heart. Expiration should not be prolonged to an extreme extent. A comfortable reserve of air in the lungs is necessary for good function of the voice.

Chewing can be used effectively to train economy of expiration. While chewing with his voice the patient is told to "shovel" air back into his mouth with his hands. In doing so he should have the feeling that the air flow is reversed. This is simpler than it sounds. The patient who used to breathe wastefully perceives the sudden slowing down of expiration with the sensation of a standstill or even the reverse of the air stream.

An even more impressive way of achieving such an effect is to go through the pantomime of eating spaghetti. Everybody remembers that persistent single strand of spaghetti that always hangs down from the mouth and has to be sucked in by strong movements of the lips (Chaplin used it once in an unforgettable scene where he mistakes a hanging-down paper streamer for his spaghetti and goes on eating it for minutes with dreamy delight). "Eating" air like spaghetti with appropriate motions of hands and lips leads even poor breathers to perfect expiration of a slow and steady stream of air.

While in general such exercises which treat the breathing act as a unit are preferable it is often necessary to strengthen neglected parts of the breathing mechanism, particularly lower chest and abdominal breathing.

Dr. G. Fairbanks (in his *Voice and Articulation Drillbook* which contains a wealth of useful hints for speech and voice exercises) recommends: place the hands, thumbs to the rear and finger tips pointing forward, on the lower ribs with firm grip; inhale against and exhale supported by the squeezing pressure.

Other useful exercises are: counting in whisper and later with full voice on expiration; reading aloud with attention to a breathing that follows elastically the natural pauses between sentences.

Dr. D. Weiss (who described the spaghetti exercise too) suggested an excellent exercise for the development of abdominal breathing: inhale deeply, steady the chest with the hands and begin to count from 121 on (each numeral has five syllables). While the attention is focused on the maintaining of chest stability abdominal breathing is used automatically and efficiently.

The main thing to remember is that lower chest and abdominal breathing should, in the end, always be a concerted function, acting as a unit. Dr. Fairbanks is right in stressing that while there is a "wrong" way of breathing that should be avoided (upper chest breathing with lifting of the shoulders for instance), there is no one single "right" way to breathe. No two persons breathe completely alike and no rigid system of breathing should be taught as a standard method.

In conclusion a word about the chances of *voice therapy*. They depend on the degree and duration of the disorder and, to a certain extent, on the age of the patient.

The earlier the misuse of the voice is diagnosed and correction begun the better the results. The younger the patient the easier the transition to improved habits of speaking and singing. In voice disorders of patients with high-quality tasks—singers and actors—everything depends on early diagnosis of a developing threat to the voice. Once it has begun to "crack" the chances for full recovery to professional use are sometimes doubtful. The same goes for pronounced disturbances of the speaking voice in patients of forty years. With all patients, prevention is worth more than the finest diagnosis; and early treatment is more promising than an attack on a fully developed disorder.

In a way, the work of the voice therapist resembles that of the restorer of fine paintings. He cannot make a Rembrandt out of a second-rate picture. But he can very often restore some of the original beauty a painting had when it left the hands of its creator.

The canvases the restorer works with show the wear and tear of time. The colors have suffered, scratches and cracks have developed, vanity has added "improvements" with new layers of paint, prudery applied a fig leaf, misguided industry contributed the false brilliancy of varnish.

Patiently the restorer works, removing useless paint here, adding a stroke with the brush there. Often he succeeds; sometimes he unveils a beauty which was not even suspected; occasionally he fails.

The human voice is such a work of art. The less one changes it, the more one respects and restores its original structure, the finer the result. The best therapy is one that restores as much as possible of the original beauty of a wonderful instrument.

XIV. *Stuttering*

In the preceding two chapters we have discussed the functional disturbances of the singing and speaking voice. Now we turn to the disorders of speech itself. The textbooks customarily treat speech and voice as separate functions of the vocal organs. Actually they belong together. In speech, voice and articulation are blended into a new unit as the chemical elements which form a new compound. For this reason, we have dealt with the normal speech along with the voice. By the same token, our discussion of functional disturbances would be incomplete without a review of the more important disorders of speech.

Speech, as we have seen before, is a very complex process. Voice (or voiceless breath) provides the raw material which is shaped by articulation into the finished product: speech sounds, words, sentences.

The centers of the brain control both the contents and the forms of speech, from a single sound to the expression of facts, ideas, emotions in the incredible variability of adult speech.

If we devote this, the first of the two concluding chapters, to stuttering we do so for a number of reasons: Stuttering is probably the best known of all speech impediments; it is very common, with adults as well as with children; it involves speech as a whole; and it is a fitting example for the discussion of many characteristic features of speech disorders.

Stuttering has been known to mankind since the dawn of history. The oldest recorded mentioning has been found on an Egyptian papyrus that dates about 2000 B.C. It contains a group of hieroglyphs which the scientists have interpreted as "hesitant speech," an expression still used sometimes as a circumscription of stuttering.

The Bible mentions speech troubles only a few times. It is doubtful whether Moses' answer to God (Exodus 4:10): "I am not a man of words . . . for I am heavy of speech and of a heavy tongue" really means stuttering or just slowness in expressing thoughts. But Isaiah (32:4) says clearly "the tongue of the stammerer shall be ready to speak plainly."

The latin word for stutterer is *balbulus*. A friend of ours, a linguist of repute, ventured an interesting interpretation of this word. The substitution of L for R is frequent in the evolution of languages (and, as we shall see, a typical speech impediment in children). Thus, balbulus might originally have been the description of a man who speaks the classic Latin of the Roman citizen like a *barbarus*, a foreigner.

Of the many famous figures in history who stuttered one even got his surname from it: Notker Balbulus, the Stammerer, a monk and writer who lived in St. Gall in Switzerland around 900 A.D. If you read Thomas Mann's latest book *The Holy Sinner* you might remember that the chronicler of this legend writes his story on Notker the Stammerer's desk.

In the English language stuttering and stammering are used as synonyms. This usage is not quite correct, but has become so generally accepted that only a purist—which we are not—will object.

For some strange reason stuttering and many other speech defects strike many people as funny. The lame, the blind can be sure of general understanding and helpfulness, but speech impediments frequently create a conflict between intentive sympathy and the instinctive reaction which makes us laugh.

If there ever was a "cruel joke" this is one. For normal speakers it is hard to realize the Hell on earth that stuttering can mean. The late Dr. J. S. Greene fought a losing battle all his life to have the "funny" stutterer banished from stage, movies and radio. He had against him a century-old tradition. Already the Italian Commedia dell' Arte, the theater of the sixteenth and seventeenth century, had with its other standardized figures (such as Arlequino, Columbina, Pantalone) the part of Tartaglia, the Stutterer, probably a great favorite with the crowds. Since then, many stuttering parts have been written for the stage. Even in opera—Wenzel in the "Bartered Bride"—stuttering has been ridiculed.

None of us—the writer included—is completely free of the sin of getting rude fun out of a stuttering joke. But, at least, we should be thoroughly ashamed of ourselves afterward.

The *incidence of stuttering* is rather high. Estimates, based on large sample statistics, run to 1½ to 2 per cent of the population. This makes it the largest single group of disabling speech defects which, according to a statistic by Dr. C. H. Voelker, affect about 3 per cent of the population.

Stuttering is about five times more frequent in males than in females. The reason for this disproportion is not quite clear. The slower speech development in boys might have something to do with it, or, as others believe, the greater preoccupation of girls with personal appearance might prevent the fixation of neurotic tendencies to the instrument of communication.

The *symptoms of stuttering* can be best understood by tracing the mechanism of their development. At the age of three to five years as many as 80 per cent of all children speak with occasional repetition of syllables called reiteration. At this point a dangerous mistake is frequently made by the parents. Instead of just overlooking the occurrence, they draw the attention of the child to it by saying: "try the difficult word again" or—even worse—by using the term stuttering in this connection. Dr. W. Johnson's "Open Letter to the Mother of a Stuttering Child" (copies available from Interstate Printers and Publishers, Danville, Illinois) gives valuable advice for the handling of this situation.

Reiteration is, to a certain extent, a perfectly normal stage in the development of speech and disappears in the vast majority of children after a while.

Only in a minority of children does this reiteration persist and increase in frequency. This symptom is called *clonus.*

After this has gone on for some time, the patient then tries to overcome his speech difficulty by applying increasing amounts of pressure. The tightly compressed lips or tongue release the built-up pressure with a sudden explosion, called *tonus.*

Finally, all kinds of *accompanying movements* are employed to conquer the steadily increasing speech difficulty: grimacing of the face muscles, movements of arms or legs, hands or feet.

What *causes* stuttering? To begin with we can dispose quickly of a false concept that should have been buried with other medieval prejudices but is still amazingly alive: that an impairment of the free motility of the tongue is to be blamed.

The small fold of mucous membrane called *frenulum* which runs from the lower surface of the tongue to the floor of the mouth has been accused of "tying the tongue." In the Gospel according to Mark (7:35) the healing of a mute is described with the words: "and the string of his tongue was loosened and he spake plain."

In the excavation of Pompeii an instrument was found, used to lift the tongue for the cutting of the frenulum. Even today, parents sometimes ask us whether an operation to "untie" the tongue would help to overcome stuttering or other speech defects.

The doctors have no reason to smile condescendingly about such layman's ignorance. One of their own ranks bears much of the responsibility for keeping alive such misconceptions. In 1841 Dr. J. F. Dieffenbach, a famous German surgeon, had the idea that an "overdevelopment" of the tongue caused stuttering and claimed to cure it by cutting a wedge-shaped piece out of the tongue. An epidemic of such operations swept the Continent and America before doctors began to realize that this procedure was just a medieval barbarism in scientific masquerade.

Although now complete agreement exists that the shape or motility of the tongue has no connection whatsoever with stuttering, other—and more serious—theories have been presented to explain stuttering in terms of organic changes. Heredity, changes in blood chemistry or metabolism, irritability of the involuntary nervous system—to mention a few—have been blamed for the development of stuttering.

Orton and Travis have stressed the development of stuttering in left-handed children who were trained to right-handed habits. They assumed that the dominance of one side of the brain—in left-handedness the right one—is interfered with by enforced shift to controlling use of the other side.

No conclusive proof could be obtained for any of these theories. Even if one finds certain physical changes associated frequently with stuttering it is difficult to determine whether these changes are a cause or a symptom of stuttering, or just co-exist with it.

On the other hand overwhelming evidence speaks for the character of *stuttering as a neurosis*: The stutterer has difficulties exclusively with sounds at the beginning or in the middle of a word. The same sound or a combination of sounds at the end of a word never presents the slightest difficulties.

Stutterers speak easily if they are alone. In the presence of people with whom they feel at ease or in generally comfortable situations they show no or only occasional symptoms of stuttering. The symptoms multiply in frequency and severity with the increase in tenseness, strangeness or hostility of a situation.

Stuttering while singing is very rare. Actors have been known to stutter heavily under ordinary circumstances but to speak perfectly normally on the stage having slipped into a different personality.

No two stutterers show the same symptoms. As a matter of fact, the amazing variability of stuttering is one of the strongest arguments against an organic cause of the impairment. The stutterer who tries to overcome the obstacles to a free flow of speech develops systems of symptoms of a complexity that betray the inventiveness of a true neurosis.

The stutterer becomes an "expert" on speech but on a faulty basis. He "knows" that a certain letter or word is "difficult"; he keeps in his mind a complicated inventory of combinations of sounds or words which have to be avoided at all costs. He is constantly preoccupied with these involved technicalities of imagined hurdles to free speech.

Stuttering is a neurotic disturbance of communication arising, as most neuroses, out of difficulties and conflicts in human relations. No single typical conflict can be described. The situations which may form the basis for the development of stuttering are as manifold as in all neuroses.

If one goes through a large number of well-investigated cases of stuttering one finds the whole gamut of conflicts that lead to neurosis: rivalry between children for affection, overprotectiveness of parents, suppressed desire, jealousy, hatred between generations and sexes, insecurity, anxiety and guilt, and the endless variety of sexual problems.

The analysts have stressed the significance of stuttering as a symptom of the repression of oral aggression. Others have blamed social conflicts as the forces that set the mechanism of the neurosis in motion.

The vast majority of stutterers develop their speech difficulties in the third or fourth year, a smaller group at the beginning of school age.

Only a minority begins to stutter in adult life, frequently in consequence of severe accidents or similar shocks. In both World Wars cases were observed of sudden stuttering which developed after severe physical or mental shocks. Such *traumatic* stuttering does not go through the stages of development we described but emerges at once with all the symptoms.

A special form of stuttering has been described by Dr. E. Froeschels as *imitation stuttering*. It is a stuttering without the inner logic of symptoms. It resembles the imitation of a stutterer by an actor or the teller of a stuttering joke. The patient goes through the motion of stuttering without exhibiting the characteristic pressure-release sequence of genuine stuttering.

On closer investigation the person can usually be identified who served as model for the imitation. In a large series of such cases the diagnosis was made only by observation of the speech symptoms, before a questioning of the patient confirmed the mechanism of imitation.

The developing of stuttering by imitation is, by the way, another reason why the portrayal of stuttering in public entertainment is not only a sin against good taste but constitutes a danger for susceptible children.

In contrast to the functional disturbances of the voice—the very existence of which is unknown to most laymen—stuttering is familiar to everybody and easy to diagnose. If still so many stutterers reach adolescence and adulthood without getting the benefit of any treatment the blame rests mostly with the patients and their relatives.

Even conscientious and affectionate parents tend to overlook fully developed speech defects in their children out of a strange mixture of resentment and guilt feelings. "He will outgrow it," they like to say in excuse for their neglect to get advice and help.

They do not realize that only a small percentage of stutterers are able to cure themselves without outside assistance. A larger group manages to live with their stuttering in a kind of armistice. By constant vigilance they are able to *conceal* the more impressive features of stuttering behind a mask of slowness and deliberation of speech. The majority of stutterers cannot come to terms with their speech impairment without some kind of expert help.

In this book we are concerned with the adult patient only. His decision to seek help for his stuttering is not made easier by the wide divergence of opinions about the right therapy he is likely to encounter.

The basic problem of the *therapy of stuttering* is: should the mechanics of stuttering be attacked or the basic neurosis itself? Or, in other words, should we treat the stuttering or the stutterer?

If one approaches this alternative from the point of view of general medical considerations one feels like deciding without hesitation in favor of a treatment that goes to the root of a condition. It goes against the grain of basic medical thinking to treat symptoms without attacking the cause of a disease.

Unfortunately, deeper insight into and wider experience with the problems of stuttering destroys, to a large extent, this simple concept.

In speaking of *psychotherapy* we think today primarily of psychoanalysis. In this connection a curious situation exists. Although analysis has staked out a theoretical claim for the treatment of stuttering as for any other neurosis, very few analysts will accept a stutterer as a patient. The very nature of stuttering puts a formidable obstacle in the path of the analytical process.

Only a few analysts have personal experience with the handling of stutterers. This and the fact that analysis is, by necessity, a time-consuming and expensive procedure exclude it from offering much practical help to the tremendous number of stutterers who need it.

But that does not settle the decision between psychotherapy and symptomatic treatment. It may be considered almost a heresy if we say that psychotherapy does not necessarily mean psychoanalysis as most people seem to believe these days. Analysis has proven its worth as one of the most powerful instruments in probing into the hidden recesses of the human mind. But there are many other ways of helping a patient to a better adjustment of his emotional conflicts. The trained psychiatrist has at his disposal a whole array of methods that can be used in approaching emotional conflicts.

The adult patient who suffers from stuttering has built up a complicated pattern of misleading and tortured reactions to "overcome" a conflict situation that was genuine in early childhood but that may have lost its meaning in the long years of its existence. Removal of the original conflict will be immediately helpful in rather recent upsets such as the stuttering after shock. It will, in no way, guarantee a satisfactory result in the stuttering of long standing. The pattern of faulty speech that, through the years, has grown into a complicated system of misguided approaches will not yield automatically when the original conflict is brought to light.

In this situation success will be more assured if the attack is directed against the disturbed pattern of speech by strengthening the forces of resistance.

If we may be permitted—in a somewhat simplified opposition to popular conceptions—to be a bit old-fashioned: the pendulum of general attitudes to psychological problems has swung too far to the side of the analytical approach. The insights and methods of analysis have opened to us countless new avenues to a better understanding of the obscurities of human emotions. But this victory over the rationalism of the nineteenth century has led to a point where *all* conflicts are being interpreted in terms of developments which are beyond the powers of the individual. People have come to believe—much to the dismay of the more thoughtful analysts—that all personal conflicts can be solved by submitting to a search of their mind as one does to an operation. They have almost forgotten the forces that lay in the personal responsibilities of each of us to face life and its conflicts with the will of resistance and character.

Psychotherapy, in any form, in the treatment of the stutterer will be, by practical necessity, in the hands of the speech therapist. In this connection, a last word of caution is needed.

Whoever undertakes psychotherapy is, in a way, in the role of a surgeon. He has to be ready to face all the implications the first step involves. The removal of an appendix is, as a rule, a simple procedure. Even ship captains and pharmacist mates have done it in an emergency. But the surgeon—and the psychotherapist—has to be ready and able to face and handle successfully any unexpected findings and situations.

Psychotherapy has become very popular. Too often it is done by persons who have no more than a rather superficial training and experience. The good that has been achieved for many patients by conscientious and expert psychotherapy has probably been outweighed by the fumbling methods of amateur psychotherapists—with or without title—who have made superficial attempts to interpret and influence the emotional conflicts of their patients.

What we said in the preceding chapter holds true with regard to speech impediments too, and to stuttering in particular. Any good speech therapy contains the element of psychotherapy. No experienced speech therapist will overlook the psychogenic background of stuttering for a moment. What use he will make of his insight into the emotional situation of his patient depends on his personal conviction and attitude.

The main task of the therapist is to convince the patient that he is perfectly able to produce normal speech. The whole complicated system of speech phobias, selective choice of words, mannerisms and body movements that the stutterer develops through the years stands and falls with his concept that speech is "difficult" for him. Whether the therapist relies on a combination of symptomatic and psychotherapeutic treatment, or whether he proceeds—as we prefer—primarily with an attack on the mechanism of stuttering, the success will always depend on the forcefulness of the therapist's persuasion of the patient to give up his faulty concept of speech.

Most of the methods that are used to lead the stutterer to a normalized use of his vocal organs are variations of a system that Klencke developed almost a hundred years ago. He began his treatments with breathing exercises and proceeded with training of the voice and finally of articulation. Special emphasis was put on relaxation.

Many systems of treatment have been built up on the basis of these recommendations. Most of the popular books of advice to stutterers employ a combination of exercises designed to relax and normalize speech production.

Since "relaxation" has become a favorite slogan, it has been made the keystone of some schools of treatment. The principle has been carried to the point where special relaxation rooms are provided to bring the stutterer into the right frame of mind.

In some systems *group therapy* has been added as a means of encouragement. Group therapy has its merits in the retraining of speech that has been lost by organic disease, for instance, with patients after a stroke or after larynx operations. In functional disturbances like stuttering it is a risky procedure. The encouragement that the patient may get from being surrounded by fellow sufferers is a deceptive one. The security that such a sympathetic atmosphere may give does not stay with the patient if he has to face normal life or hostile situations. In addition, there is considerable danger that the stutterer, with the adaptability of the neurotic, might pick up new mannerisms of stuttering speech from other patients.

Dr. A. Liebmann whom we mentioned before as one of the fathers of modern speech therapy employed the *drawling method.* He taught the patient to overcome the speech block by prolongation of the vowels and the use of a slow and steady rhythm of speech. The method is still useful in the treatment of small children or in cases where other methods have failed.

The *chewing method* which we described in the preceding chapter is particularly suited to the treatment of stuttering. It is there that the method has found the widest acceptance.

It permits the patient to make a completely new start in his approach to speech. By explaining to the patient the chewing approach in the way we described in the preceding chapter it is usually not difficult to convey to him the idea that he has at his disposal a "natural" way of speaking, quite different from the "wrong" way he has used so far.

It is very impressive to witness the first interview with a stutterer to whom the chewing idea is offered. The patient who stuttered heavily in the tense atmosphere of the first encounter with the therapist is suddenly able to produce bits of unimpeded speech with the help of the chewing motions.

The critical phase of the treatment comes sometime later when the patient has to learn to *accept* permanently the free speech, offered and demonstrated to him by the method. The resistance of the neurosis against dismissal on short notice emerges when the patient is asked to employ the chewing approach in every day's free speech.

The situation that develops is familiar to everybody who has experience with the treatment of neurotics. The patient finds all kinds of excuses to interrupt treatment; he may ridicule the methods or exhibit hostility toward the therapist.

It is at this point that the energy and patience of the therapist and his ability to handle the mechanics of neurosis decide the outcome. He must employ all the resources of his personality to keep alive the conviction of the patient that free speech is at his disposal and to strengthen the resolution of the patient to conquer his speech impediment by his own effort.

As an interesting commentary we might mention in passing the opinion of an experienced analyst who felt that the success of the chewing approach could be interpreted as opening an active outlet in speech for the aggressive tendencies of the stutterer.

The main advantage of the chewing method lies in the appeal to an inborn function which is easily available and never disturbed by the destructive forces of the neurosis. The method has been used on a great many patients with good and permanent results by a number of therapists.

We have discussed stuttering as the classical example of a functional speech defect at some length. It gave us the opportunity to study many of the problems we encounter in speech therapy.

In the next, the concluding chapter of this book, we shall deal more summarily with other impairments of speech.

XV. *Other Speech Disturbances*

As numerous as the elements that go into speech are the disorders that may beset it. To describe them all would disrupt the framework of this book. It is not written for the professional speech therapist who can turn to one of the many good textbooks that are available to him. To give you an idea of speech disorders and a better understanding of the problems that arise in their diagnosis and treatment, it will suffice to select typical examples of the more important forms of disturbed speech.

To draw a sharp line between normal and defective speech is not always possible. Is the ideal the normal, or is normal what the average person does? When we discussed the disorders of the speaking voice we had already occasion to raise this question. Hardly anybody speaks with an ideal voice; most people exhibit some deviation from what the expert would consider perfect production.

By the same token, nobody speaks "normally" in every respect. Place or country of origin, social standing, education, work, age and many other factors put their stamp on speech, create numerous variations from ideal usage.

When we discussed the imprint of the personality on the speaking voice (Chapter V) we saw how far the deviations from the "norm" may go that character traits and emotional changes can produce.

Take, for instance, the case of overfast or overslow speech. We find *tachylalia* (Greek for fast speech) on both ends of the scale of speech temperament, with the highly intelligent who thinks extremely fast and with the thoughtless chatterbox or, to quote Shakespeare, with the gentleman "that loves to hear himself talk, and will speak more in a minute than he will stand to in a month." Likewise *bradylalia*, the overslow manner of speech, may be the expression of dull-wittedness, or of careful weighing of each word, or of an arrogance that tries to enforce attention by a slow diction.

In such conditions the borders between normal and abnormal speech are very fluid. In a given case of tachylalia we can use the social function of speech as a yardstick and consider the intelligibility of the overfast speech. If the speed reaches the limit where it interferes with easy understanding the borderline of normalcy has been crossed and the realm of speech disorders has been entered.

To slow down the fast speaker is not easy. One good method that has been used with success is to make the patient aware of his speech movements. It is like changing the automatic action of fast walking into a conscious succession of single movements of feet and legs. By continuing exercises along these lines for a while one may succeed in creating a new, slower pattern of speech.

Intelligibility is, of course, of no use in judging the abnormalcy of slow speech because there is no problem to understand the speaker. Here we have to rely, more or less, on esthetic considerations. Excessive slowness and hesitation of speech creates in the listener an almot painful impression, an impatient desire to urge the speaker on to faster delivery. The abnormal character of bradylalia becomes more obvious if the speaker intersperses his speech—sometimes before each word—with meaningless vowel-like utterances ("a-a").

To speed up the pattern of overslow speech is very difficult and often impossible. Too deep are the roots of this mannerism in the personality of the speaker to permit an easy change by outside influence.

Tachylalia is frequently a symptom of a more general disorder of speech, called *cluttering*. It is a counterpart to stuttering, in that it changes the whole pattern of speech. But while stuttering is a well-known disturbance of speech, cluttering, although very frequent, has remained a kind of stepchild in the public knowledge of speech disorders.

The scientific name for cluttering, *tumultus sermonis*, the tumult of speech, is a good description of the speech pattern of the clutterer. Both the child and the adult who clutter are persons that, figuratively speaking, fall constantly over their own feet. They speak very fast but without precision. They do not finish sentences, they distort syllables, they make mistakes of articulation to the point of unintelligibility.

In contrast to the stutterer who suffers severely from his speech impediment the clutterer is blissfully ignorant of his hasty and blurred pattern of speech. While the stutterer encounters more difficulties if he focuses his attention on his speech, the clutterer improves with greater concentration. His personality is characterized by lack of attention, poor memory, general hastiness and restlessness.

At the bottom of cluttering lies a disparity between thinking and speaking. The clutterer has a very strong drive to express his, often turbulent, thoughts in speech, but he is trapped by the mechanics of speaking and gets lost in the middle of words and sentences.

The same happens to the clutterer in reading. Many of these patients had reading difficulties in school which might have persisted in later years. They jump over syllables, words and even lines, and find it hard to give a detailed account of what they just read.

The memory of the clutterer for words is generally poor, which has led some researchers to assume an organic defect in brain development as the cause of cluttering. They point to the fact that cluttering occurs frequently in some families as another proof of an organic basis of cluttering. But the research that has been done in this direction has not yet produced conclusive proof for this assumption.

As different as cluttering and stuttering are, they are not so rarely found in the same patient, with cluttering forming the basis on which later stuttering develops.

Although the incidence of cluttering is rather high, much less is known about its background in terms of personality problems than in the case of stuttering, because too few clutterers seek the help of the doctor or speech therapist.

Cluttering is one of the speech impediments that are frequently neglected. The patient, whether child or adult, is not much aware of it. Parents like to overlook it. Even if the child is hard to understand, the mother, with her possessive instinct, goes to great length to assume and maintain the part of the interpreter who "translates" to others the meaning of the child's turbulent and garbled speech. The adult clutterer seeks help only if he experiences difficulties in his chosen work.

In contrast to the handling of stuttering, the *treatment of cluttering* is designed to improve attention to the structure and mechanics of speaking. Exercises of details of articulation, reading practice with emphasis to single words, training of attention, memory and concentration, underscoring of speech movements are the elements around which the therapy is built. Patience and energy, both of the therapist and the patient, are needed. No fast results can be expected.

So far, we have discussed only such disorders which change the whole pattern of speech. Another, rather frequent, occurrence is the *disturbance* of single elements *of articulation.* Speech sounds can be affected in many ways. The patient may either distort or mispronounce certain speech sounds, he may omit speech sounds completely, or he may substitute speech sounds for intended ones. One or more of the three zones of articulation can be involved, and all possible combinations of defective articulation occur.

A typical example of distortion of a speech sound is the *lisping* which involves the S sound (S, Sh, Z). If you watch the speech of other people with an attentive ear you will be astonished how often you hear a more or less pronounced lisp.

Lisping may be connected with dental abnormalities but in the majority of cases no visible organic changes can be found in the speaking organs.

Speech therapists classify lisping according to the positions of the tongue in speaking the S. If the tip of the tongue presses against the edges of the upper incisor teeth it is called *addental* lisp. If the tip of the tongue protrudes between the teeth it is an *interdental* lisp. In both cases instead of the S a fricative Th is produced. In a third form, the *lateral* lisp, one side of the tongue is raised more vigorously or is pressed against the molar teeth. Air then escapes into the cheek.

In the treatment of lisping, as of most other distortions of articulation, it is important to understand that the patient usually does *not* hear his own speech defect. Parents, teachers often try to correct mistakes of articulation by loud and exaggerated demonstration of the correct sound with the exhortation "say it right." The poor victim of this well-meant but rather mistaken therapy tries hard to imitate the example. He is firmly convinced that he produces a sound exactly like the one that is offered to him but still employs the old defective articulation.

To break this pattern, acoustic suggestions alone are useless. The therapist has to direct the attention of the patient to the proper position and the motions of lips, teeth, tongue in producing a given sound. This cannot always be achieved directly, particularly with children who are hardly conscious of speech movements. Manipulations of all kinds must be employed to get the desired effect. The "tricks" which are used to produce all speech sounds in a patient are important tools of the speech therapist.

When the speech sound is properly performed for the first time without any distortion the tedious work begins of establishing this new pattern as a habit to replace the wrong manner that has been used for many years.

Parents, patients, even teachers are frequently impatient with the speech therapist whom they suspect of prolonging his treatments for earthly gains. They have the idea that all that is needed to correct a defective speech is to demonstrate the proper usage. Even with an intelligent and willing patient—not always the rule—it takes often a lot of time to steer him through the period of adaptation, of back-sliding and discouragement, of slow gains, to final victory. Habits of years die hard, and new patterns are established only by constant repetition and practice under expert supervision.

We mentioned already one typical substitution of sound: the replacement of R by L. Many such substitutions are observed, sometimes accumulating to the degree that speech becomes unintelligible.

One of the reasons for these and other defects of articulation is *impaired hearing*. Congenital deafness or loss of hearing before the completion of full development of speech interferes excessively with the ability to articulate clearly; even loss of hearing in later years may influence articulation. The loss of hearing of the high frequencies is particularly deleterious because the fricatives (S, Sh, F, V, Th, Z, H) are normally spoken at high levels and are not heard in this type of deafness.

To teach deaf patients to speak is a great art requiring tremendous patience, ingenuity, practical psychology and the ability to gain and hold the confidence of the patient.

The same holds true of severe disorders of the speaking mechanism. An impressive example of such a condition is the speech treatment in *cerebral palsy*. Here we deal with a disturbance of the controlling power of the motor centers of the brain in consequence of damage during pregnancy or during the act of birth.

Although cerebral palsy is common (according to Dr. M. F. Evans in ½ per cent of all births) it has been, for a long time, a stepchild of medicine. Until about twenty years ago, these unfortunate patients, with their severe disturbances of general muscular co-ordination, were considered as feeble-minded persons for whom little or nothing could be done.

When doctors and teachers began to study cerebral palsy patients, it was found that frequently behind the motor imbalance and speech impairment an average or, sometimes, even a high intelligence is hidden.

One of these patients, Dr. E. R. Carlson, has written a very moving book *Born That Way* in which he described his own breaking out of the prison of twitching muscles and his fight against tremendous odds that transformed a helpless cripple into a prominent doctor. It is in the training of the patient with cerebral palsy where modern speech therapy finds one of its greatest triumphs.

Difficulties of articulation may arise from a *foreign language background*. Aside from imperfections in melody and rhythm, foreign accent is essentially an articulatory problem. Some speech sounds exist only in one language (such as the Th or the Wh in English). Others are spoken with a different mechanism. The foreign born has a tendency to hang on to the production of speech sounds used in the old language while speaking the new one. His ear may be reliable in discerning his own accent in the mouths of others but does not help him to spot his own mistakes. He is shocked to "hear" his accent for the first time if he listens to a recording of his speech.

To correct such accent is possible in children and adolescents for whom it is relatively simple to establish new patterns of the mechanics of speech sounds and of melody and rhythm of speech. It is next to impossible with the adult who may be able to eliminate his more glaring mistakes but who is set in his speaking ways by half a lifetime of habits of speech movements, of melody and rhythm of speech.

It has been argued that a *bilingual background* may be damaging to the speech development of children and liable to produce speech disorders. In this connection, we agree with Dr. C. Van Riper's thoughtful commentary. He feels that not bilingualism but poor general speech environment—so frequently associated with bilingual background—is the source of speech difficulties. He believes that children who have grown up in an atmosphere of refined speech habits and who have learned two languages at the same time seem to have rather benefited by this experience.

A special group of articulatory disturbances are the *disorders of nasal resonance*. In Chapter IV we have seen that all sounds of the English language, except M, N, Ng, are spoken with the elevated soft palate that prevents air from flowing into the nose.

If this palatal elevation and closure does not function properly speech will assume a strong *nasality*. The plosive sounds (P B D T G K) cannot be produced properly or at all. We call this condition *hyperrhinolalia*. While some of these cases have a functional basis, the majority is of organic origin. Some diseases, like infantile paralysis or diphtheria may produce a paralysis of the soft palate. Scars of the soft palate from poorly done operations of tonsils and adenoids may interfere with palatal action.

The best known example of excessive hyperrhinolalia is the speech of the *cleft palate* patient. During embryonal development the hard and soft palate are formed in separate structures on both sides which meet and fuse in the mid-line. If this fusion remains imperfect, cleft palate results. That happens—according to Dr. O. L. Backus—in about one in every thousand to twelve hundred of all births.

Aside from the impairment of speech cleft palate may interfere with drinking and eating. As we have seen, in the act of swallowing the soft palate seals off the nose and prevents food from entering the nose. The defect of the cleft palate leaves the nose without this protection, and regurgitation of fluid into the nose makes the feeding of the infant difficult.

To cover the defect by plastic surgery a number of ingenious operations have been devised. The results are not always satisfactory. The pull of the palatal muscles on the delicate sutures is a danger to the undisturbed healing of the united palate. And even if it remains intact the speech may still be nasal because the newly formed palate is too short to perfect complete closure on elevation.

Where operation is not feasible or advisable, or where surgery has resulted in failure, another method is used. The defect can be covered by so-called obturators, plastic plates that are individually molded and attached to the upper teeth by dental work.

The cleft palate patient goes through life with a severe handicap. Aside from the direct consequences of impaired communication in school and work, the psychological implications are tremendous. To feel rejected as part of a minority group is hard enough but made tolerable because of the comradeship with others in the same group. A severe speech defect is a heavy individual burden. A person who has to live with such a stigma in the midst of normal people is isolated by his defect. The rejection that too frequently is felt is the harder to take because of the thoughtless indifference or even ridicule that normal people offer to patients with speech defects.

Lately, more attention has been paid to the rehabilitation of cleft palate patients. Hospitals and speech centers have formed special teams of surgeons, pediatricians, speech therapists, psychiatrists, to bring effective help to cleft palate cases. There the chances of operative procedures or of covering of the defect by obturators can be weighed, training of the muscles of palate and throat conducted by various exercises under expert supervision and the personality problems handled.

The opposite of hyperrhinolalia is the *lack of nasality*, called *hyporhinolalia*. In this condition the passage of air which is needed to produce nasal sounds is blocked by contraction of the soft palate or by some obstacle in the nasopharynx or in the nose. The most frequent cause of such blockage is the presence of *adenoids* in the nasopharynx, but impairment of free nasal breathing by nasal polyps or excessive deviations of the nasal septum may produce the same effect.

Temporary blockage of the nose by swelling of the mucous membranes in colds, sinus troubles, allergies may reduce the nasal resonance, up to the degree of complete lack of nasality.

Hyporhinolalia is characterized by a muffled type of speech. You can produce it by compressing your nostrils with thumb and index finger. The treatment of hyporhinolalia is essentially medical: removing of adenoids or polyps, correction of the septum, clearing of nasal infections, management of allergies.

At this point we should like to remind you of our discussion in Chapter V of the changes of nasal resonance under the influence of emotional imbalances. Any increase or decrease of the congestion of the nasal membranes, any variation in the tonus of the palatal muscles, that occurs under the impact of moods and tensions, will produce varying degrees of hyper- or hyponasality of speech. The observation of such changes gives valuable clues to the emotional profile of a patient.

Speech, as we have seen at the end of Chapter IV, is controlled by the centers of the brain. If one or a combination of these centers is damaged severe impairment of the speech faculties results. We call this reduced capacity of speech, due to brain lesion, *aphasia* (Greek for speechlessness). The aphasic patient may have normal and well-functioning vocal organs but the "executive" part of speech production is disrupted.

Such a brain defect may be congenital, due to imperfections of brain development before birth. In the adult who slowly or suddenly develops severe disturbances of speech control, the aphasia indicates a damage to brain centers by disease. Brain tumors, for instance, may produce speech defects as the first symptom if they press on a speech center.

The best known example of sudden aphasia is the loss of speech caused by a *stroke*. In a stroke, a blood vessel of the brain bursts and the blood that cannot escape from the closed and tightly packed space inside the skull presses as a clot on the cortex of the brain.

Together with other parts of the brain that control the motion of arms and legs the speech centers may be involved. As we have seen, these centers are, in most people, located in the left half of the brain that controls the right side of the body. Therefore, loss of speech is more frequent in patients with muscular paralysis of the right side.

The type of aphasia that results depends on the location of the damage. If the pressure has hurt Broca's motor center the patient cannot perform the motor act of speaking any more. He understands anything he hears, he can read or think in words but cannot express his thoughts in spoken words.

Damage to other centers may produce a wide range of symptoms: inability to name objects, amnesia of all degrees, difficulties in reading and writing or in understanding of speech, interference with the associative powers of the brain.

The study of these aphasias is of great importance to neurologists and speech therapists alike. Most of our knowledge of brain function derives from the analysis of the symptoms of localized brain injuries. Many patients owe their life to the early diagnosis of the exact location of a brain tumor by the symptoms of deficient function which made successful operation possible.

By the same token, the treatment of aphasias, caused by a stroke, has been immensely helped by a better understanding of the mechanics of brain function. The speech training of these patients has become an important part of their general rehabilitation.

In former years the unfortunate victims of a stroke were left to an existence that was too often no better than being buried alive. Today, teams of neurologists, physical therapists, speech therapists and social workers have developed methods for the rehabilitation of the aphasic. It is a very slow process and the results depend, after the reversibility of the brain damage, both on the knowledge of the therapist and the courage and will power of the patient. But, at least, hope can be offered where quiet despair used to reign.

We have now reached the end of our discussions and we feel that we should say good-by to you who have stayed with us so long.

Custom has it that the author of a book on a scientific subject should speak to the reader only through the medium of the facts he presents. A doctor who writes for lay readers stands somewhere between the scientist and the professional writer. He may be forgiven for a personal word of parting.

We have to confess that we face with regret the ending of the quiet hours of writing. In our civilization which abounds with so much loneliness in the midst of crowds, writing is one of the few pursuits where a man may be alone without being lonely.

We were in your company. We thought of you as a patient who wants the answers—he so seldom gets—to his many questions. The longer our discussions went on the more you became, in our imagination, a good friend with whom one is used to talk things over, without hurry and hesitation, in frankness and fellowship. We hope that our conversations were mutually profitable.

As to ourselves, we know they were. One of the incidental gains of medical writing for lay readers is that the author is forced to go back to many of the sources he studied through the years and to clarify to himself many details that became obscure. And he acquires a fresh overall view of his field which will enrich his daily tasks.

As for you, we are reasonably sure that our discussions will be of practical use, making it easier for you to give better care to your voice, in health as well as in disease.

Beyond that, we hope that you will lay this book aside with deep admiration for the genius of creation that produced the wonderful instrument of the human voice, equally suited to mirror all the emotions of man in song and to express the richness of the mind in speech.

Essentially, both song and speech are nothing but sounding breath. The rhythm of breathing that sustains life from birth to the hour of death becomes, through song and speech, the precious achievement that lifts human beings high over all other forms of organic life.

With the instinct of a great poet Goethe has chosen the tidal rhythm of breathing as a symbol of man's indebtedness to life and creator:

> Two graces are given us while we breathe:
> To take in air, to unload it with ease.
> The one oppresses, the other relieves;
> Life so wondrous a mixture achieves.
> You thank the Lord for pressure and strain,
> And thank him when he releases you again.

Recommendations for Further Reading

THE READER WHO DESIRES TO GET MORE INFORMATION ON THE subjects of this book is advised to consult one of the books or papers on this list. The selection of these sources—out of the tremendous wealth of logopedic literature—was made with the idea in mind to recommend such publications that present sufficient detail in an authoritative and readable form. Of course, such recommendation does not mean endorsement of all opinions expressed in these books and papers. But at this point of his studies the reader is on his own and has to form his personal opinions.

V. E. Negus, Comparative Anatomy and Physiology of the Larynx. Grune and Stratton, 1949.
A survey of the development of the larynx through the animal kingdom, from the amphibians to man (with a large number of illustrations).

Robert Curry, The Mechanism of the Human Voice. Longmans, Green & Company, 1940.
Out of print but available in larger libraries. A study of all important research on structure and function of the vocal organs. Particularly valuable because of very complete bibliography.

Charles A. Culver, Musical Acoustics. Blakiston, 1951.
A standard textbook on all phases of musical acoustics, com-

prehensively written in an easy-readable style, profusely illustrated.

Robert West, Lou Kennedy, Anna Carr, The Rehabilitation of Speech. Harper & Brothers, 1947.
A standard textbook on speech and voice disturbances, diagnosis and therapy.

Wendell Johnson, Speech Problems of Children. Grune and Stratton, 1950.
The disturbances of speech are discussed in a popular manner by a number of leading speech therapists.

Emil Froeschels, Twentieth Century Speech and Voice Correction. Philosophical Library, 1948.
A group of outstanding therapists discusses newer advances in speech and voice therapy.

Deso A. Weiss and Helen Beebe, The Chewing Approach to Speech and Voice Therapy. S. Karger, 1951.
A collection of articles by a number of speech and voice therapists who relate their experiences with the chewing method.

Grant Fairbanks, Voice and Articulation Drillbook. Harper & Brothers, 1940.
A system of practical exercises for all components of speech and voice. Very useful for everybody who does speech and voice therapy.

Special studies of general interest are contained in the following papers (which may be consulted in any good medical library):

Joel J. Pressman, "Physiology of the Vocal Cords in Phonation and Respiration." *Archives of Otolaryngology*, March, 1942.
A detailed study of the anatomy and function of the vocal cords, with numerous illustrations (referred to in Chapter III).

Paul J. Moses, "Vocal Analysis." *Archives of Otolaryngology*, August, 1948.

A study of the connections between voice and personality (referred to in Chapter V).

Deso A. Weiss, "The Pubertal Change of the Human Voice (Mutation)." *Folia Phoniatrica*, Vol. 2, No. 3, 1950.
A survey of the physiology and the disturbances of the change of voice (referred to in Chapter XII).

The *Journal of Speech and Hearing Disorders*, published by the American Speech and Hearing Association, should be consulted for recent developments in the field.

Index

Set in Linotype Janson
Format by Edwin H. Kaplin
Manufactured by The Haddon Craftsmen, Inc.
Published by HARPER & BROTHERS, *New York*